Easy Delicious Gluten-Free One-Pot Meals

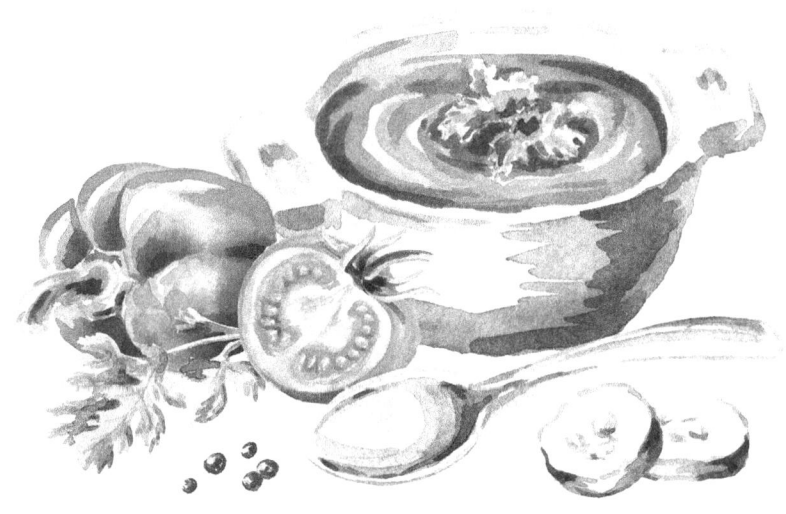

Julie Cameron

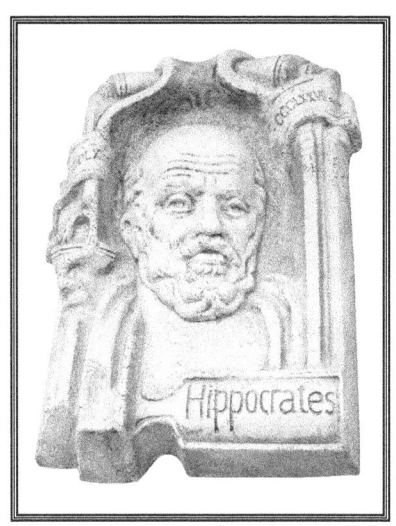

"Let food be thy medicine and medicine be thy food."

"The natural healing force within each of us is the greatest force in getting well."

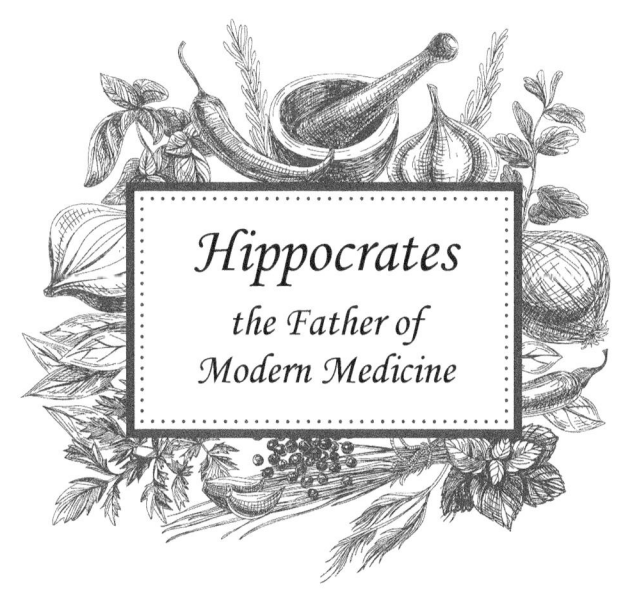

Hippocrates
the Father of Modern Medicine

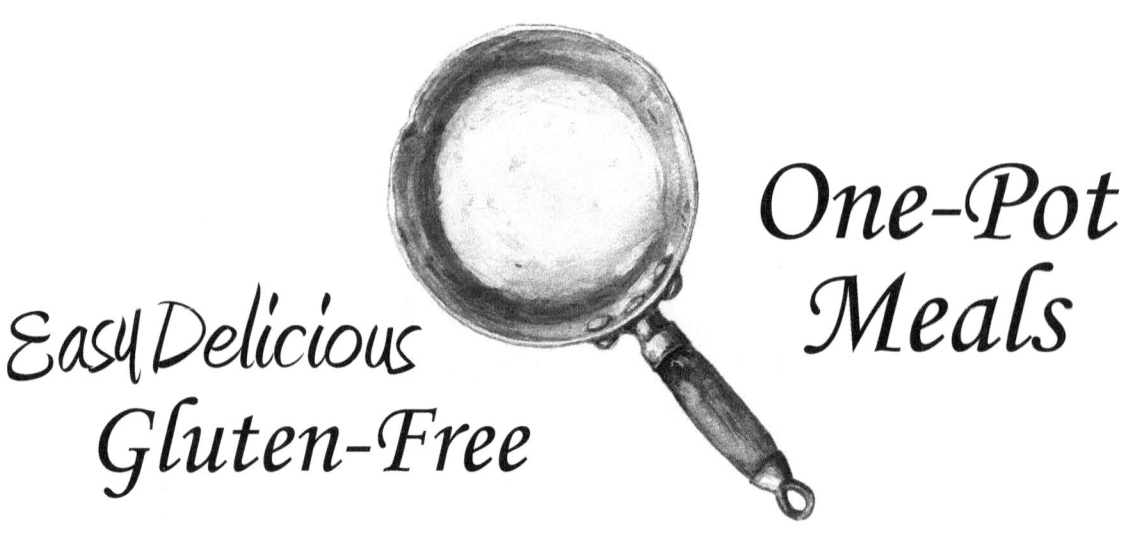

Easy Delicious Gluten-Free One-Pot Meals

Copyright © 2019 by Julie Cameron

All Rights Reserved

No part of this book may be reproduced in any form by any means without the prior written permission of the Publisher except for brief quotes used in literary reviews.

Published in the United States of America by
Easy Delicious Gluten-Free
visit us at
Easy Gluten-Free Cooking
www.easygfcooking.com

ISBN-13: 978-0-9997923-2-2

Suggested Library of Congress Cataloging-in-Publication Data

Cameron, Julie

Easy Delicious Gluten-Free One-Pot Meals

/ Julie Cameron

1. Gluten-free diet--Recipes.   2. Quick and easy cooking.   3. One-dish meals.

This cookbook is for informational purposes only. Its content is not meant to be a substitute for professional medical advice, diagnosis, or treatment. Always seek the advice of a qualified healthcare provider with regards to your health or the health of those you are responsible for.

First Edition

*This cookbook is dedicated to all
the gluten-free people around the world.
I hope that you enjoy these recipes
and I hope that they help you
to regain good health.*

- Julie Cameron -

*Special thanks to my husband Kevin,
the Official Taste Tester,
who lovingly and patiently supported me
while I wrote this cookbook.*

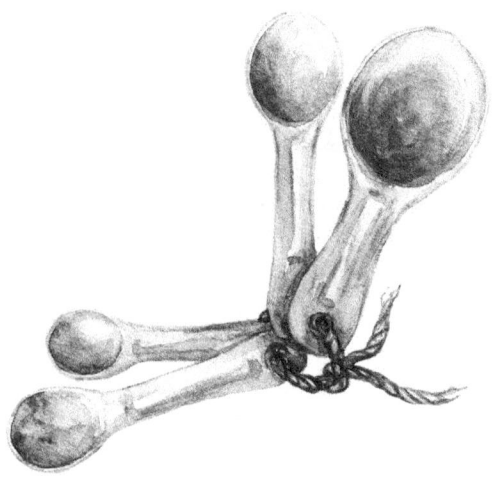

Table of Contents

1   Introduction
7   What is gluten?
11   Where is gluten found?
15   What foods are safe to eat?
29   Reading food labels
37   Testing for gluten intolerance
43   Cookware and utensils
51   Converted rice
53   Measuring pasta
57   Tips
63   Beef and Lamb Recipes
95   Chicken Recipes
121   Pork Recipes
153   Seafood Recipes
169   Vegetarian Recipes
188   Photo Credits

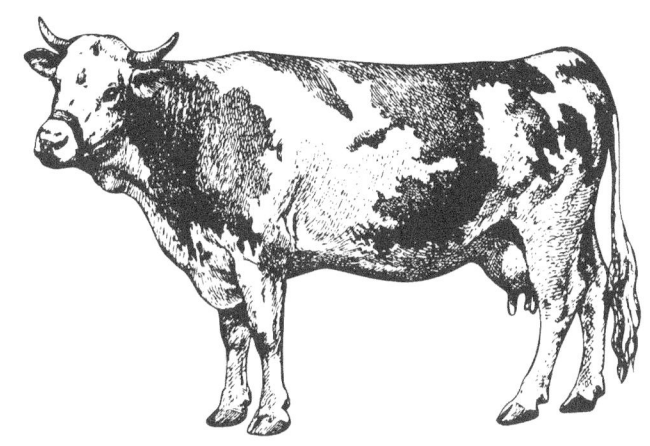

Beef and Lamb Recipes

Meals in a Skillet

64   Taco in a Skillet
65   Beefy Italian Skillet
66   Chili Macaroni Skillet
67   Asian Beef and Broccoli Skillet
68   Hungarian Goulash Skillet
69   Original Hamburger Macaroni Skillet
70   Greek Skillet with Olives and Feta
71   Salisbury Beef and Mushroom Skillet
72   Mexican Beef and Rice Skillet
73   Cheeseburger Macaroni Skillet
74   Beef Stew in a Skillet
75   Stroganoff Mushroom Skillet
76   Skillet Shepherd's Pie
78   Skillet Tamale Pie

Soups and Stews

80   Savory Beef Stew with Winter Vegetables
81   Classic Beef Chili
82   Gluten-Free Cornbread Muffins
84   Easy Vegetable Beef Soup
85   Saucy Cabbage and Hamburger Soup
86   October Cider Stew
87   Herbed French (Italian) Onion Soup
88   Mediterranean Lamb Stew
89   Stuffed Pepper Soup
90   Easy Vietnamese Pho
92   Hot and Smoky Beer and Bacon Chili
93   Herbed Provencal Beef Stew

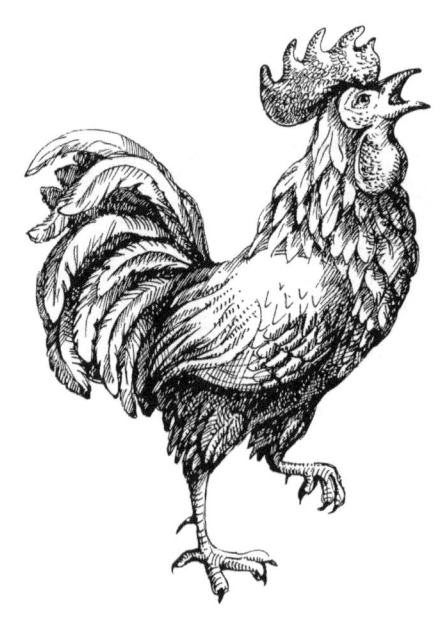

Chicken Recipes

Meals in a Skillet

- 96 Southwest Fajita Skillet
- 97 Tandoori Chicken Skillet
- 98 Chicken Curry Skillet
- 99 Cheesy Chicken and Rice Skillet
- 100 Chicken Broccoli Alfredo Skillet
- 101 Stovetop Chicken Tetrazzini
- 102 Chipotle Chicken and Rice

Soups and Stews

- 104 Classic Chicken Noodle Soup
- 105 White Bean Chili with Chicken and Red Onion
- 106 California Rancho Posole
- 107 Chicken and Rice Soup
- 108 Southwestern Chicken Stew
- 110 Chicken and Vegetable Bean Soup
- 111 Santa Fe Soup
- 112 Chicken and Summer Vegetable Stew
- 114 Moroccan Chicken and Apricot Stew
- 116 Italian Hunter's Chicken
- 118 Chunky Cream of Chicken and Mushroom Soup
- 119 Jalapeno Chicken and Rice Stew

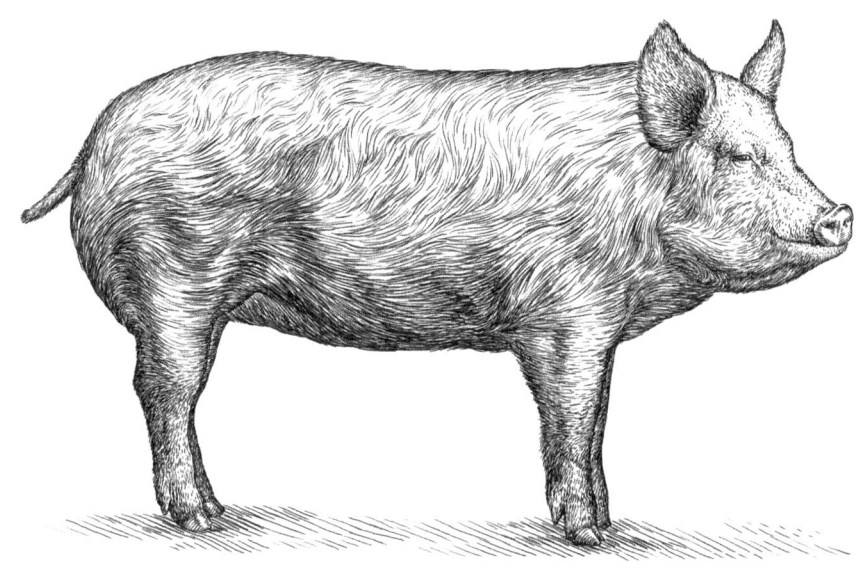

Pork Recipes

Meals in a Skillet

- 122 Creole Rice Skillet
- 123 Spanish Paella Skillet
- 124 Tastes Like Ravioli Skillet
- 125 Creamy Mushroom and Ham Skillet
- 126 Zesty Sausage, Potato, and Pepper Skillet
- 127 Hoppin' John
- 128 Skillet Red Beans and Rice with Spicy Sausage
- 130 Spanish Catalan Potato Skillet
- 131 Skillet Scalloped Potatoes and Ham with Mushrooms
- 132 Spaghetti Amatrice
- 133 Jammin' Jambalaya

Soups and Stews

- 134 Split Pea and Ham Soup
- 136 Winter Pork Stew with Smoked Paprika
- 138 Mexican Pork Chili Verde Stew
- 139 Italian White Bean, Ham, and Rosemary Soup
- 140 Spicy Sausage and Kale Soup
- 142 Fall Dinner Ham and Potato Soup
- 143 Easy French Cassoulet
- 144 Hearty Minestrone Soup in a Flash
- 146 Best Ever Pizza Soup
- 148 Tuscan Sausage and Bean Soup
- 150 Minnesota Wild Rice Soup
- 152 Spicy Chorizo Corn Chowder

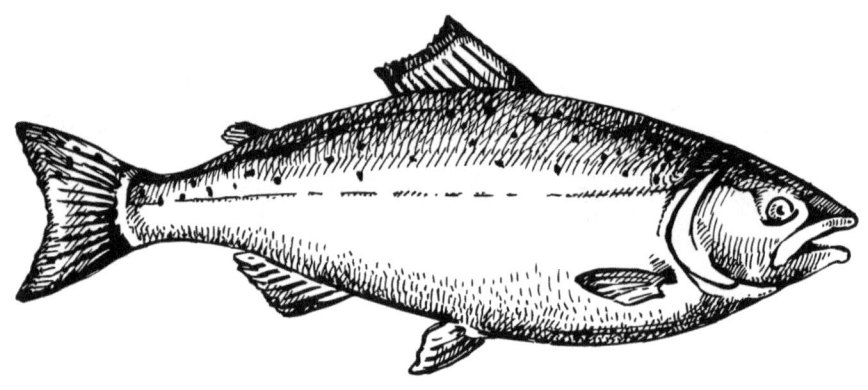

Seafood Recipes

Meals in a Skillet

154 Cheesy Salmon Skillet
155 Tasty Tuna Macaroni Skillet
156 Tuna Mushroom Skillet

Soups and Stews

157 New England Clam Chowder
158 Herbed Salmon Chowder
160 Manhattan Clam Chowder
161 Chipotle Shrimp and Avocado Soup
162 Easy Cioppino
164 Thai Shrimp and Noodle Soup
166 Shrimp and Rice Gumbo

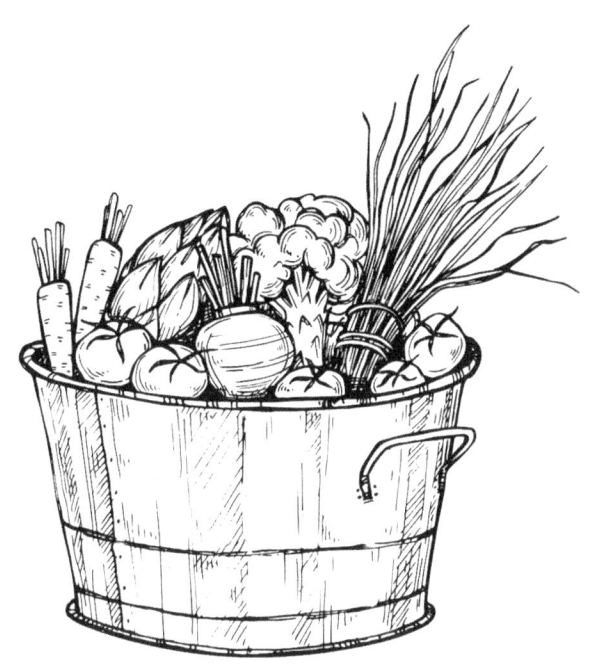

Vegetarian Recipes

Meals in a Skillet

- 170   Pasta Primavera Skillet
- 171   Butternut Squash and Parmesan Skillet
- 172   Lentils with Kale and Sweet Potatoes

Soups and Stews

- 173   Provencal White Bean and Tomato Stew
- 174   Summertime Gazpacho
- 176   Sweet Potato and Black Bean Chili
- 177   Herbed Tomato Soup
- 178   Easy Ratatouille
- 180   Turkish Spinach and Lentil Stew
- 181   Savory Mushroom and Lentil Stew
- 182   Sweet Apple and Cabbage Stew
- 183   Winter Squash and Apple Soup
- 184   Italian Vegetable Stew
- 186   Curry Spiced Lentils

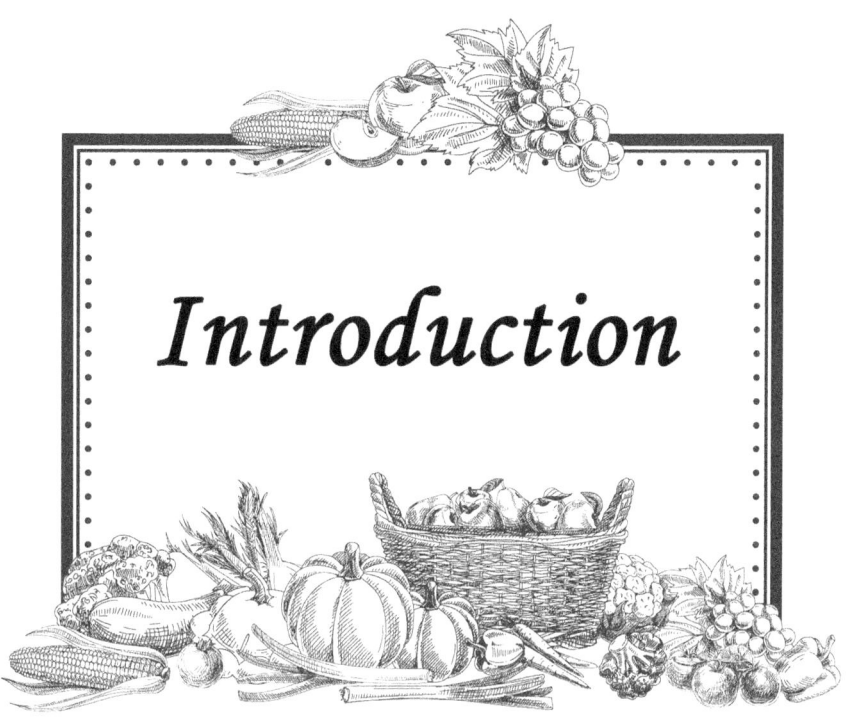

Introduction

Congratulations on making the commitment to feel better and live a healthier life by cooking gluten-free.

I have been cooking gluten-free for over 15 years and if I can learn to do it so can you.

I spent most of my life in poor health due to gluten intolerance. Then in September of 2001 everything changed. My husband and I took a trip to Paris and the south of France to celebrate a special wedding anniversary.

During the trip my lifelong symptoms of bloating, stomachache, diarrhea, and fatigue greatly diminished while eating a traditional Provençal diet that is low in wheat. Wheat is a grain that contains gluten.

After returning home I told my doctor that my health had been good for the first time in a long time. He dismissed it as a result of not being under stress while on vacation.

In reality the trip had been extremely stressful as it had coincided with the September 11, 2001 terrorist attacks during which close friends and family members were affected.

Despite the stress my health improved significantly while eating the vegetables, lean meats, and beans that were the staples of the Provençal diet – a diet where bread and wheat products are optional.

I knew something else was wrong – that my symptoms weren't just the result of stress in my life. My intuition was right. I sought out a new doctor who drew samples of blood and tested for food intolerances. The tests flagged possible problems with gluten which is a protein found in wheat, barley, and rye.

Additional testing for gluten intolerance via a simple and inexpensive genetic test confirmed that I had a genetic predisposition to the inability to tolerate gluten.

After removing gluten from my diet my symptoms disappeared and have not returned in over 15 years. The exceptions have been a handful of incidents where gluten had been unknowingly introduced into my food.

It is possible to get your life back

If you are suffering from symptoms of gluten intolerance then following a gluten-free diet may help you regain good health.

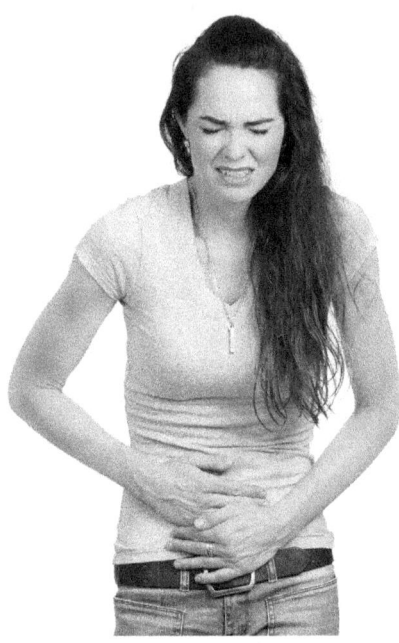

You don't have to feel this way

Different people exhibit different symptoms when their digestive tract is exposed to gluten. For those who are not gluten intolerant no symptoms will appear. For those who are gluten intolerant there are varying levels of discomfort that depend on how gluten intolerant the individual is.

Like autism, gluten intolerance lies along a spectrum where the mildly gluten intolerant may have barely noticeable symptoms (foggy mental state, easily fatigued) while those who react strongly to gluten may experience severe symptoms such as violent diarrhea and severe abdominal pain.

Common Symptoms of Gluten Intolerance

Gastrointestinal

- Diarrhea
- Intestinal gas / bloating
- Abdominal pain / cramping
- Constipation

Mental

- Depression
- Foggy mental state
- Inability to concentrate
- Headaches

Overall Health

- Chronic fatigue
- Unexplained acute weight loss (in severe cases where intestinal damage has occurred)
- Weight gain (bloating and retention of fluids due to reaction to gluten)
- Bone or joint pain
- Unexplained infertility in women
- Short stature
- Failure to thrive in children
- Poor hair growth
- Lackluster skin and nails

Consult with your doctor to be sure

If you suspect you or a family member has gluten intolerance then it is very important that you consult with your doctor to rule out other health problems which may cause similar symptoms.

Your doctor may want to test for Celiac Disease which is diagnosed by confirming damage to your intestinal tract caused by the consumption of gluten-containing foods.

Intestinal damage can be confirmed via a relatively painless procedure called an endoscopy where a flexible endoscope is inserted into your intestinal tract. The endoscope takes digital photographic images that can reveal intestinal damage.

Some specialized endoscopes have robotic tips that can pinch a small biopsy sample that can be further studied by your doctor. If your symptoms are severe your doctor may want to do additional testing to further assess the level of damage. Advanced cases of Celiac Disease have been linked with intestinal cancer so it is important to talk to your doctor.

It is possible to suffer from symptoms of gluten intolerance without having Celiac Disease. If your doctor suggests an endoscopy do not be afraid. It is relatively painless and low risk. Most insurance plans cover diagnostic procedures such as endoscopy so do not hesitate if you think that the cost will be prohibitive – your health is worth it.

An ounce of prevention is worth a pound of cure

The best way to keep gluten intolerance from progressing to Celiac Disease and possibly cancer is to follow the gluten-free diet for life. Removing gluten from your diet will help prevent intestinal damage if you are gluten intolerant.

There are no adverse side effects to removing gluten from your diet so rest assured that a gluten-free diet can be a safe, positive choice for you and your family.

Just like quitting smoking, the minute that those who are gluten intolerant remove gluten from their diet is the minute that their bodies begin to heal.

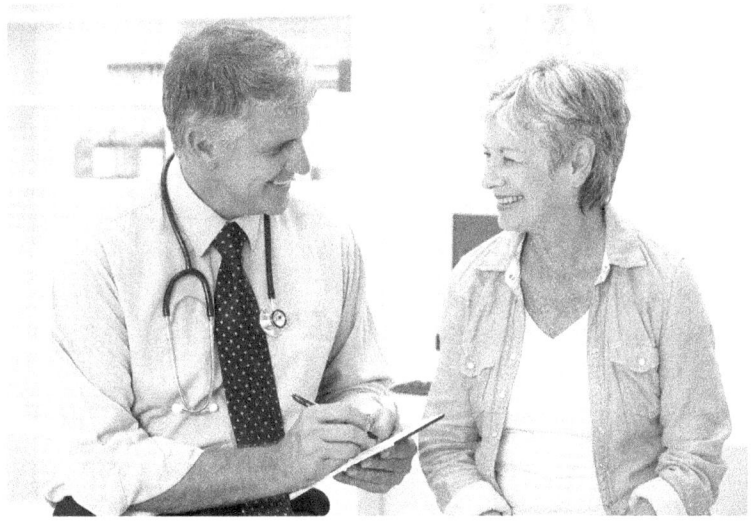

Always consult with your doctor to be sure

You are not alone in this

Take comfort in knowing that if you are gluten intolerant you are in good company. Gluten intolerance is one of the most common genetic conditions. It affects at least 1 in every 100 people and can be more common depending upon ancestry.

Ironically, those of Italian descent have a higher incidence of gluten intolerance. The Italian diet features an abundance of delicious gluten-containing pastas. Italians who cannot eat pasta have adapted by enjoying dishes made from beans (fagioli), corn (polenta), or rice (risotto). Many restaurants in Italy offer gluten-free pastas made from rice or corn – a dining trend that is catching on in the United States.

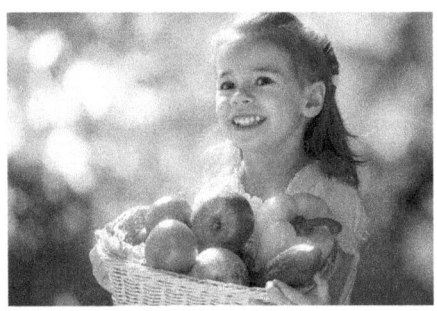

As worldwide awareness of gluten intolerance grows those of us who must adopt a gluten-free diet will have an easier time finding foods that are safe for us, when we travel and when we shop in our grocery store or eat out in restaurants.

The good news is that the treatment for gluten intolerance is entirely within your control.

Adopting a gluten-free diet for life will relieve you of your current gastrointestinal symptoms and may help prevent intestinal damage, Celiac Disease, and intestinal cancers.

Take the first step

You will be pleasantly surprised to find that cooking gluten-free is not difficult once you know the rules.

The recipes in this cookbook were chosen from my personal recipes developed over the last fifteen years. They have been optimized for ease of preparation, minimum time to table, and use of 'safe' processed foods for convenience.

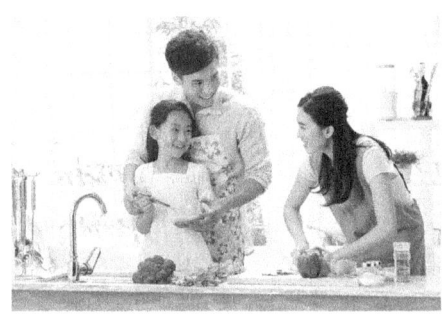

Cooking gluten-free is not difficult if you know the rules

These recipes use low-cost, readily-available ingredients. If you are like me, then crème fraîche is probably not in your refrigerator, lobster is probably not in your budget, and you probably don't have a lot of time to prepare dinner.

These recipes are easy, inexpensive, and designed to make use of the naturally gluten-free foods you already have in your pantry and your refrigerator.

> *Most of the ingredients used in these recipes are already in your pantry or refrigerator.*

Relax - you only need to make small changes in how you shop for groceries

You may have heard that it is difficult to find foods that are gluten-free. This is only true if the foods are processed foods.

Most unprocessed foods are naturally gluten-free. This cookbook will teach you how to use more unprocessed foods in your diet and how to identify whether a processed food is safe for you to eat.

There is no need to buy special flours or special mixes. No specialized cooking equipment is required to prepare these recipes.

When you know what foods are 'safe' then cooking gluten-free need not be difficult or expensive.

This cookbook contains information on choosing gluten-free foods and learning how to prepare them without contaminating them with gluten-containing foods you may have in your kitchen (cross-contamination).

Anyone can learn to cook gluten-free

These recipes have been written to provide extra instruction to ensure that even beginner cooks (including older children) can cook them successfully.

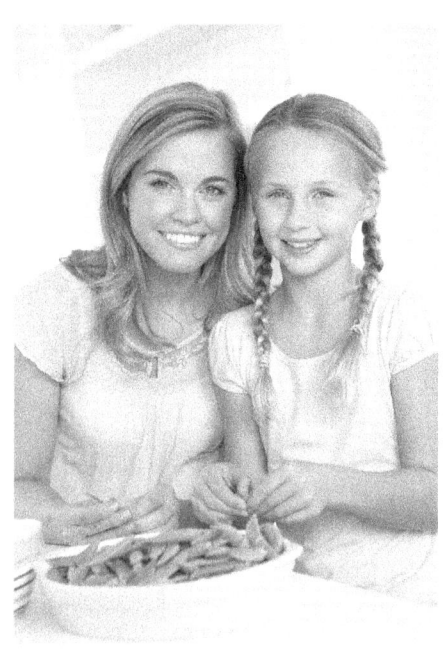

Cooking is fun when you have good instructions

Don't worry if you have no experience cooking or you think that you are capable of 'burning water'.

All of these recipes are easy, delicious, and best of all they're gluten-free.

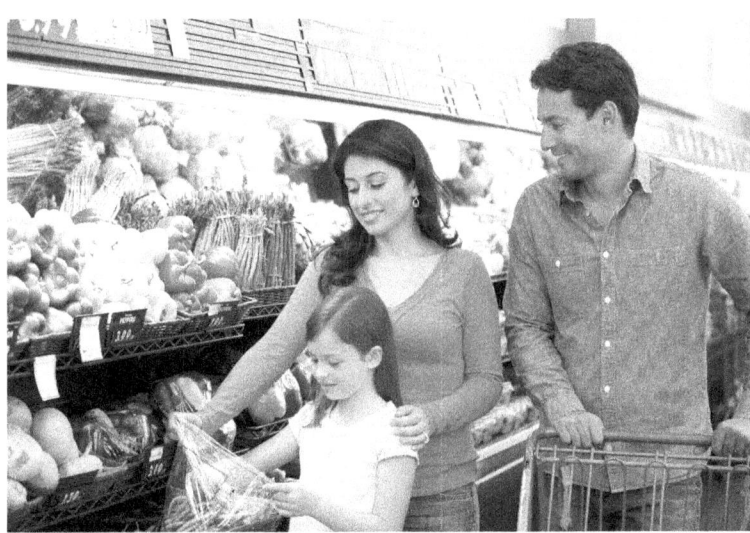

Shopping gluten-free isn't difficult if you know the rules

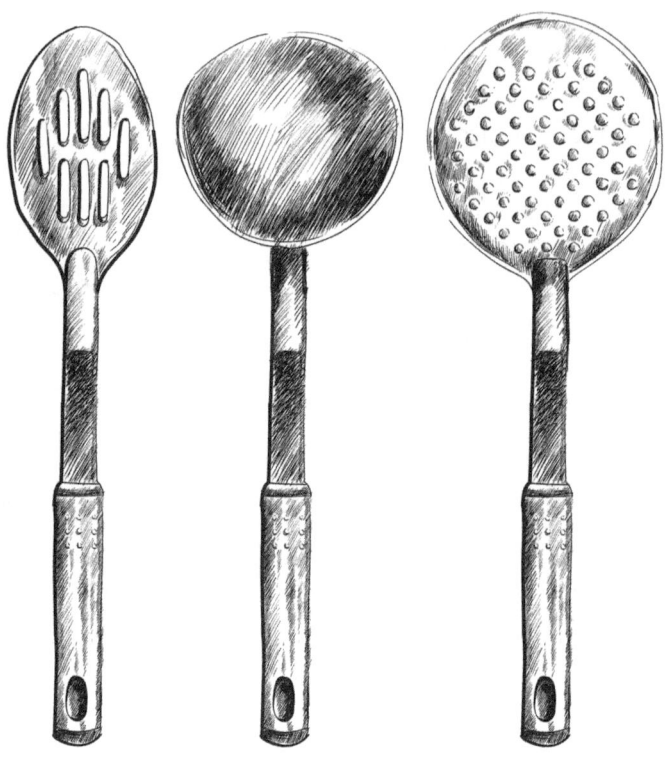

What is gluten?

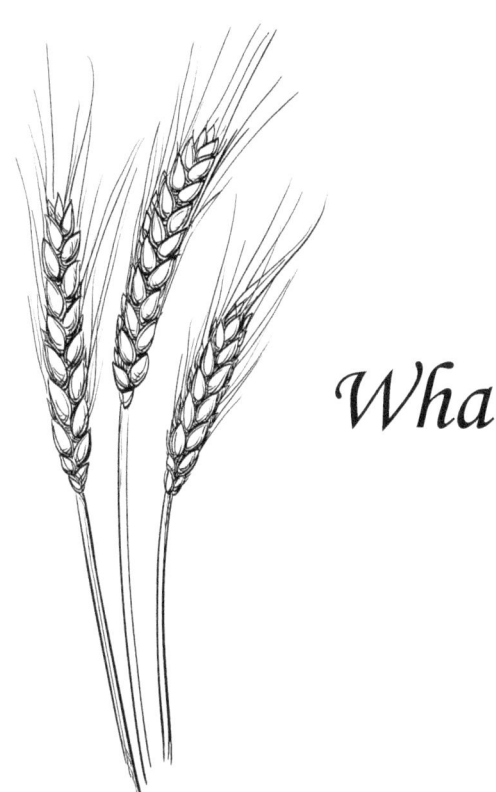

At its most basic definition gluten is a protein that consists of a combination of two component proteins, gliadin and glutenin.

Gluten occurs naturally in the grains wheat, barley, and rye.

Foods made with wheat, barley, and rye will contain gluten. This includes most pasta, breads, cakes, and many desserts.

Processed foods that are made using the ground flours of wheat, barley, and rye will also contain gluten.

Some alcoholic beverages such as beer that is made from barley and whiskey that is made from rye will contain small amounts of gluten.

Those who are gluten intolerant need to remove gluten from their diet or they will risk intestinal damage.

Do not despair. There are gluten-free grains that can be substituted for wheat, barley, and rye.

You will still be able to enjoy pasta, breads, cakes, desserts, and even a (gluten-free) beer.

Once you know what foods are safe to eat and what foods you need to find a gluten-free substitute for then you will be able to eat almost anything you normally eat - including pizza, lasagna, macaroni and cheese, spaghetti, pancakes, grilled cheese sandwiches, cakes, English muffins, and cookies.

> *There are gluten-free foods that can be substituted for almost every food that contains gluten.*

What does gluten look like?

Gluten is the sticky substance easily identified in unbaked bread and pizza dough. Gluten is what gives dough its elasticity and ability to stretch when you knead it.

It is also the substance that gives baked bread its spongy 'spring'. This springy structure can be approximated in gluten-free products by using an additive called xanthan gum.

Adopting a gluten-free diet has never been easier. Nearly all foods that normally contain gluten - including pasta - can be made without gluten-containing ingredients.

The key to adhering to a gluten-free diet is learning to identify which foods contain gluten and learning to read product labels to identify if there are any gluten-containing ingredients. Then you can either buy a gluten-free substitute or cook your own gluten-free version of the food.

Why is gluten harmful?

The same sticky substance (gluten) that makes bread dough stick to your fingers also has the capacity to irritate your intestinal tract.

For some people this causes no problem. For those who are gluten intolerant the gluten causes inflammation and an immunological response that can be compared to a mild allergic reaction.

Over time this low-level inflammation can damage your intestines (Celiac Disease) and in severe cases it can lead to cancer.

To give an easily understandable analogy consider that there are some people who come in contact with poison ivy and do not develop itchy red skin and blisters.

Similarly, a person who is not gluten intolerant will not exhibit symptoms such as diarrhea and stomachache when they eat foods that contain wheat, barley, and rye.

This person is among the lucky majority of the population who may continue to eat 'regular' cakes, cookies, pastas, and breads without worry or harm.

On the other side of the spectrum is the person who brushes up against poison ivy and breaks out in swelling, hives, and itchy blisters. This person is highly sensitive to poison ivy in a similar way that those who are gluten intolerant are highly sensitive to gluten.

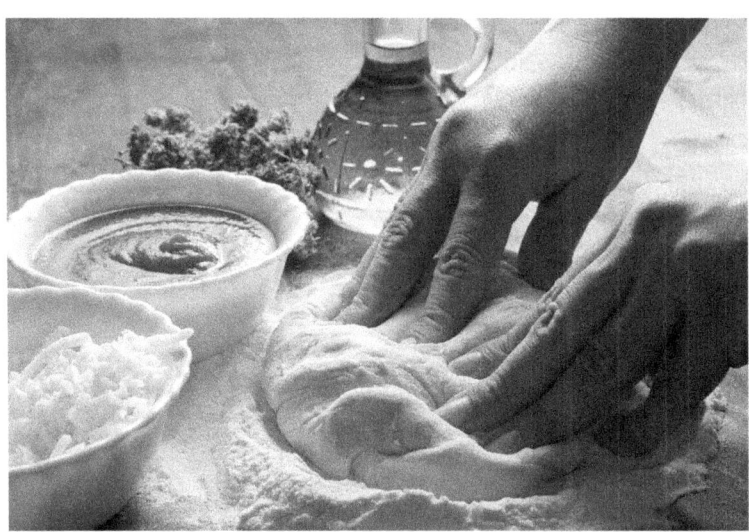

Gluten gives dough the ability to stretch

For the small but significant portion of the population who are gluten intolerant it is essential that they remove gluten from their diet or they will risk intestinal damage.

Why is gluten intolerance not well known?

In the United States the word is finally getting out about gluten intolerance. Despite being a world leader in technology and other industries Americans are playing catch up when it comes to education about gluten.

Many countries in Scandinavia and Europe have long recognized the disabling effects of being sensitive to gluten. Gluten intolerance is given the same respect and regard as Americans give to peanut allergies.

In many European countries children who exhibit symptoms of gluten intolerance are tested at an early age for gluten sensitivity to avoid life-long cumulative intestinal damage.

Because the prevalence of gluten intolerance in Italy is relatively high it is respected for the medical condition that it is.

Italian drugstores (farmacia) carry gluten-free breads, pasta, and other gluten-free foods on the pharmacy shelves.

Just like Americans consider antibiotics and other pharmaceutical drugs 'medically necessary' the Italians rightly consider gluten-free foods to be medicine that is necessary for good health.

People think my symptoms are 'in my head'

It hurts when others don't take our suffering seriously - especially those who are closest to us such as family and friends. And make no mistake about it, if you are gluten intolerant and haven't yet removed gluten from your diet you are suffering.

From minor symptoms such as inability to concentrate to disabling conditions such as severe diarrhea that keeps you 'never far from a restroom' to life-changing consequences such as infertility and miscarriage it is clear that those who are gluten intolerant suffer greatly - up to and including facing the life-threatening prospect of intestinal cancer.

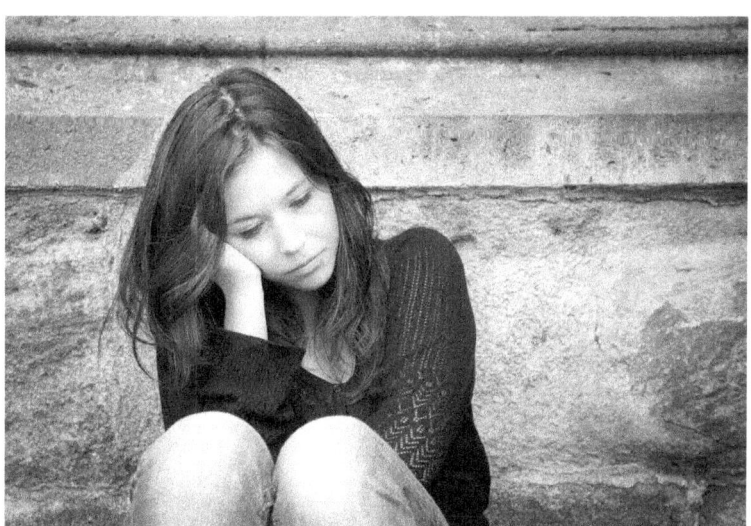

Depression can be a symptom of gluten intolerance

If you are gluten intolerant then you are probably a brave person who suffers in silence.

It isn't that your family and friends don't care that you suffer; it is simply a matter of them not understanding how you suffer.

The outside world can see the suffering caused by an allergic reaction to poison ivy because the sufferer's symptoms are largely external (blisters, hives).

Because the symptoms of gluten intolerance are largely internal (diarrhea, intestinal pain) it is more difficult for others to see the suffering that the gluten intolerant endure.

To further compound the misery, many of the symptoms of gluten intolerance are embarrassing (intestinal gas, diarrhea) or intensely private (depression, infertility).

It is not surprising that those who suffer from these symptoms are not always eager to share the details of their suffering.

As such, awareness of gluten intolerance is not as high as it should be. Many people go undiagnosed for years until their suffering is so great that their friends, family, and even their doctors finally take them seriously and they finally get the help they need.

So don't give up. Find a sympathetic health care professional who can get to the root of your symptoms and accurately diagnose whether you suffer from gluten intolerance or another health issue.

If you are diagnosed as gluten intolerant then learn as much as you can about avoiding gluten. Make a resolve to adopt a gluten-free diet for life.

There is currently no 'cure' for gluten intolerance but by avoiding gluten for life your body will begin to heal and you can expect to live a reasonably normal, healthy life.

Isn't the extra effort that is required to prepare gluten-free meals a small price to pay for the ability to enjoy your retirement years in good health, surrounded by family and friends?

You owe it to yourself and those you love to be there for the future – both yours and theirs.

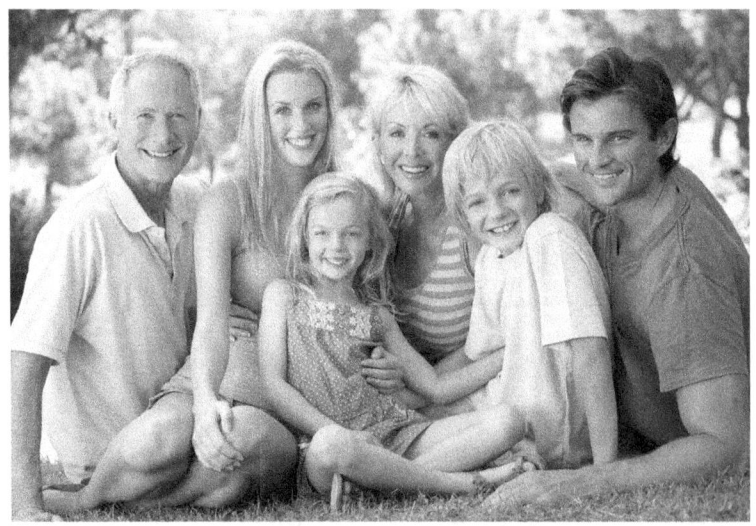

*Be there for those you love
- adopt a gluten-free diet for life*

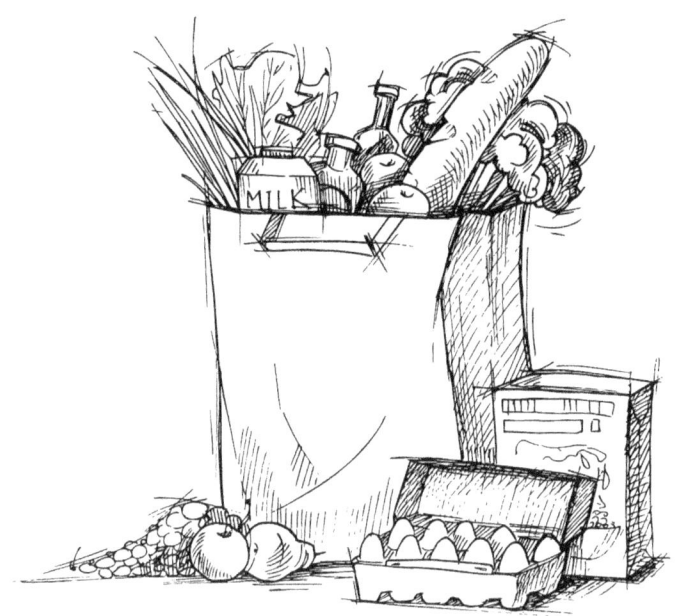

Where is gluten found?

Many people who are diagnosed with gluten intolerance worry that they won't be able to find anything to eat. Gluten is in many foods, especially processed and convenience foods.

There is no need to fear. There are many foods that are naturally gluten-free and you will have plenty to eat. Furthermore, foods that are naturally gluten-free are often nutritious and good for your health.

This cookbook will show you how to avoid gluten in your diet and how to substitute gluten-free ingredients in recipes so that you can easily prepare delicious, nutritious gluten-free meals in your home.

Gluten is found in wheat products

Wheat and the products made from it will contain gluten.

Gluten is found in most breads, cookies, cakes, pizza, pasta, breakfast cereals, gravies, and processed foods that use wheat to flavor or thicken them.

See the section on **Reading Food Labels** for help in determining if processed foods contain gluten.

Many dishes made from wheat flour can be made 'safe' by substituting flours from naturally gluten-free foods such as rice, corn, potatoes, tapioca, sorghum, millet, and uncontaminated oats that are certified as gluten-free.

Many grocery stores now carry gluten-free breads and baked goods. These gluten-free products are often stocked in the refrigerator or freezer sections to prolong product life.

At some well-stocked grocers it is even possible to find refrigerated or frozen gluten-free pie crust, bread dough, and cookie dough.

Those who must follow the gluten-free diet have even more options including the option of using a baking mix to make their own baked goods. In addition to specialty manufacturers of gluten-free baking mixes many mainstream manufacturers have begun to offer gluten-free baking mixes.

Consumers can find a variety of gluten-free baking mixes for cakes, cookies, brownies, and pizza crust. To top it off (literally) several manufacturers of ready-to-use cake frostings have changed their recipes to use ingredients that do not contain gluten.

So don't worry - if you are gluten intolerant you can still have your cake and eat it too.

For those who love pasta there are gluten-free pastas made from rice and corn that are nearly identical in appearance, taste, and texture to pastas made from wheat.

You don't have to give up bread, cakes, cookies, and pasta. All it takes is a little effort to identify which products are safe for you to consume. For help in determining if products contain gluten refer to the section titled **Reading Food Labels**.

Gluten is found in barley products

For some, the hardest part of adhering to the gluten-free diet is giving up a favorite food or beverage. When I found out I couldn't eat 'regular' pizza I quickly learned how to find gluten-free pizza crust mixes and pre-made gluten-free crusts to make my own pizza at home.

Then I found out about beer. Most beers contain barley and as one doctor so eloquently stated: 'beer is liquid gluten'. I resigned myself to the fact that I was going to have to drink root beer (which is gluten-free) on Friday Pizza Night.

I was wrong. I didn't have to give up beer. There are several manufacturers that offer gluten-free beers that are made from sorghum, corn, millet, or rice.

There are also 'gluten-reduced' beers that have been manufactured using an enzyme that reduces the gluten to below 20 parts per million (ppm) which is a threshold set by the United States Food and Drug Administration (USFDA). This threshold is generally believed to be the minimum amount of gluten that induces symptoms in those who are gluten intolerant.

For many this threshold is acceptable and they can enjoy 'gluten-reduced' beers. If you are highly sensitive you may not be able to tolerate even this very small amount of gluten so you will need to choose a beer that is labeled 'gluten-free'.

Barley is also used in soups and stews, some types of hard liquor, and it can be an ingredient in breads so check product labels carefully.

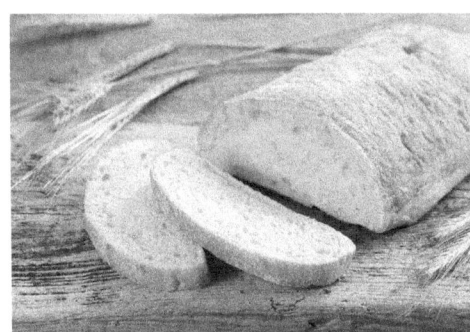

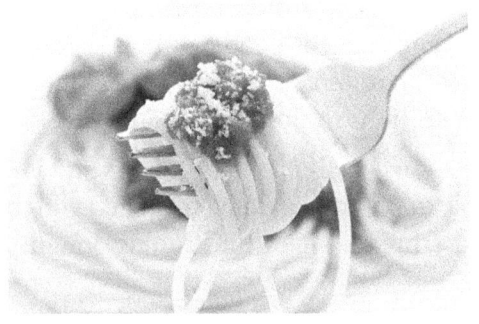

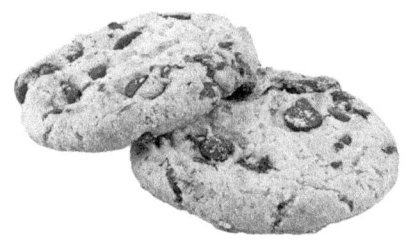

Many processed foods are made with wheat flour

Gluten is found in rye products

Rye is a gluten-containing grain that is most commonly used in hearty breads. It is relatively easy to identify as an ingredient because the rye flour colors the bread a rich brown.

Rye is also used as an ingredient in distilled liquors such as vodka, whiskey, and bourbon. There is some debate as to whether the distilling process adequately removes gluten from the liquor.

Even when all gluten has been removed during the distilling process some distilled liquors can still be unsafe for the gluten intolerant. Additives such as Caramel Coloring (often made from wheat) can reintroduce gluten after the distilling process.

Some people find that they can tolerate distilled liquors while others cannot. As always, if you experience symptoms of gluten intolerance when consuming distilled liquors do not continue to consume them.

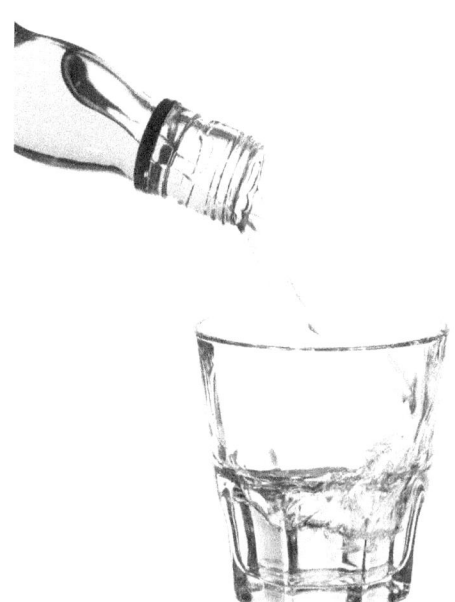

Whiskey made from rye may contain residual gluten

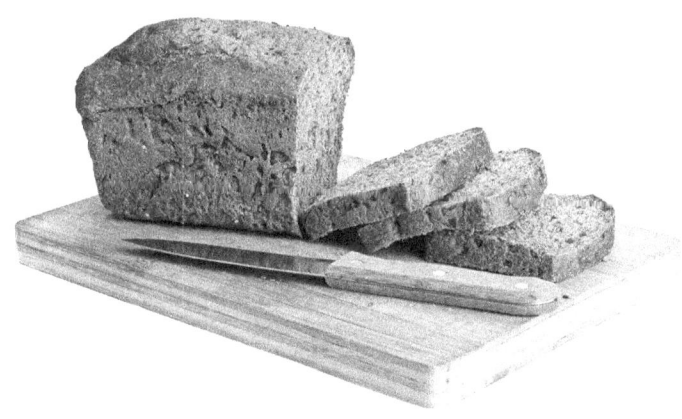

Rye bread contains gluten

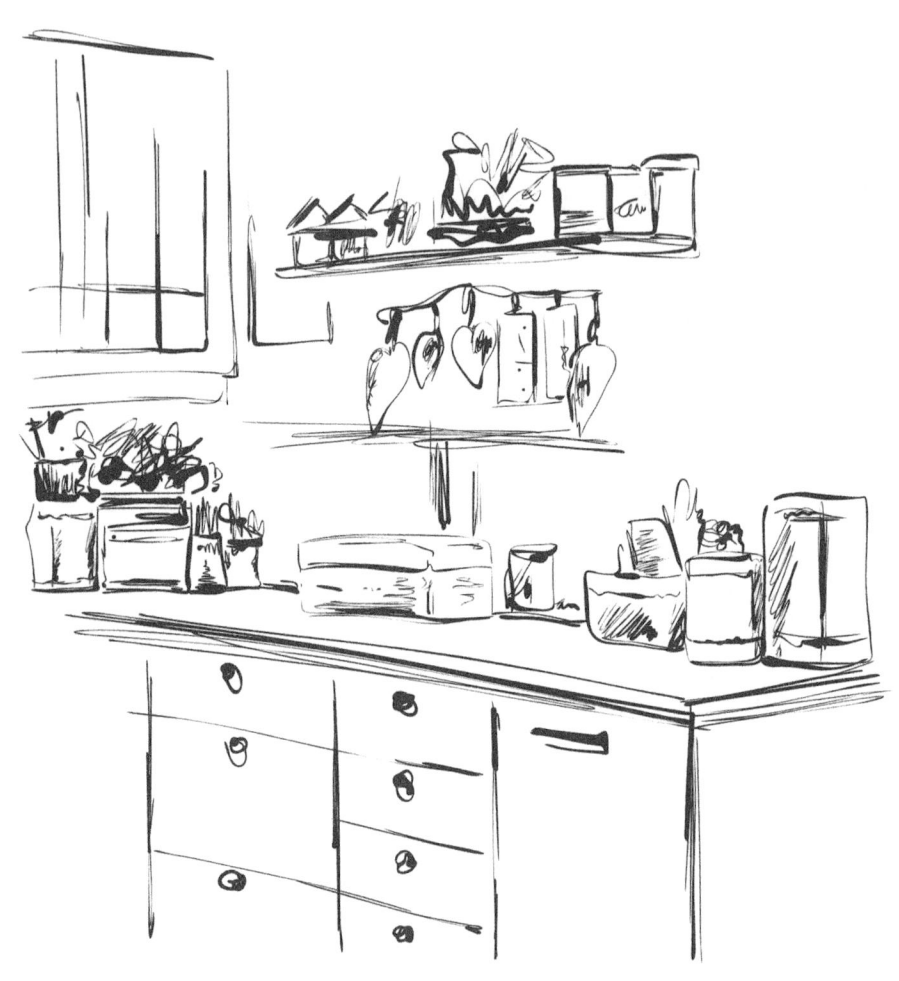

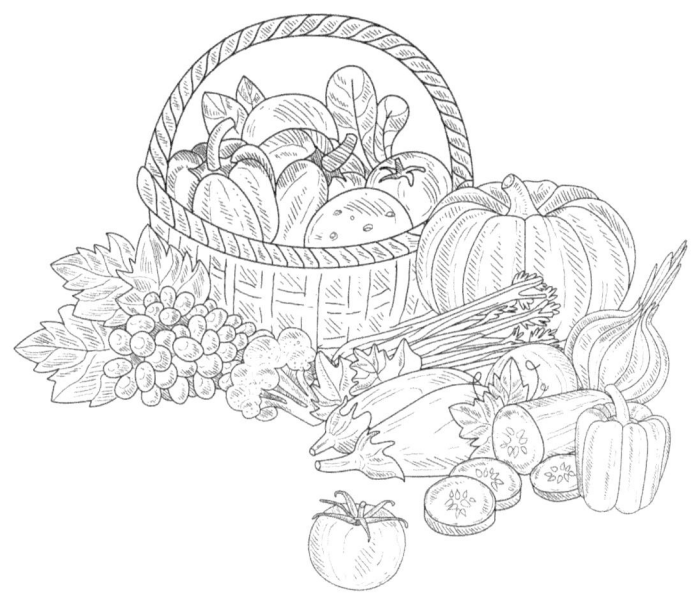

What foods are safe to eat?

Even if you can't eat foods that contain wheat, barley, or rye there are still a lot of foods that you can eat. Most unprocessed foods are safe to eat as long as they don't contain or have not been contaminated with wheat, barley, or rye.

Processed and unprocessed foods

For our purposes we will define an unprocessed food as food that is in its native form without additional ingredients or additives. Examples of unprocessed foods are strawberries picked from the vine, a chicken breast that was skinned and deboned by your butcher, or a glass of milk.

Unprocessed foods are native, original foods. They may have been washed (packaged lettuce), cut (celery sticks), peeled (butternut squash), chopped (mixed fruits in a fruit bowl), skinned and/or deboned (chicken), or pasteurized (milk) but no new ingredients have intentionally been added in the process of packaging the food for consumption.

Many unprocessed foods are located in the outer perimeter of your supermarket in the produce, dairy, and meat sections. Unprocessed foods often have a short shelf life and require refrigeration to remain fresh.

For our purposes any food to which additional ingredients have intentionally been added is a processed food. Examples of processed foods are strawberry jam (strawberries), chicken nuggets (chicken), and ice cream (milk).

Processed foods offer convenience because they allow busy cooks to skip preparation steps that are done by the manufacturer. An example of this time-saving convenience is opening a can of chicken noodle soup versus making the soup 'from scratch'.

Manufacturers often convert an unprocessed food to a processed food to increase shelf life without the need to refrigerate the food.

Processing methods can include canning (fruit, tuna, tomatoes), drying and/or powdering (powdered milk, dried herbs and spices, mashed potato flakes, dried beans), or the addition of preservatives (pickles, hard salami, some processed 'loaf' and 'jar' cheeses).

Most processed foods are located in the inner aisles of your grocery store because they usually do not require refrigeration.

Consumption of processed foods can potentially be unsafe for the gluten intolerant. Gluten-containing ingredients can either intentionally be added (such as wheat-based noodles in chicken noodle soup) or the processed food can unintentionally be contaminated with gluten (such as oatmeal contaminated with wheat flour during milling).

Naturally gluten-free foods

There are many unprocessed foods that are naturally gluten-free. The following is an abbreviated listing of unprocessed foods that are generally safe for consumption by those who are gluten intolerant.

Vegetables

All vegetables are naturally gluten-free.

Eat as much as you want of unprocessed artichoke, asparagus, beets, bell pepper, Bok Choy, broccoli, Brussels sprouts, cabbage, carrots, cauliflower, celery, corn, cucumbers, eggplant, fennel, garlic, green beans, green peas, hot peppers, kale, leeks, lettuce, okra, onions, parsnips, potatoes, radishes, shallots, sweet potatoes, pumpkin, rutabaga, spinach, Swiss chard, tomatillo, tomato, turnips, winter squash, yams, zucchini, and other vegetables.

When it comes to vegetables the rule is simple: if you can grow it in your garden you can eat it on your plate (as long as it's unprocessed).

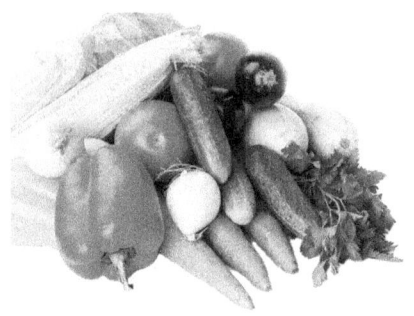

All vegetables are naturally gluten-free

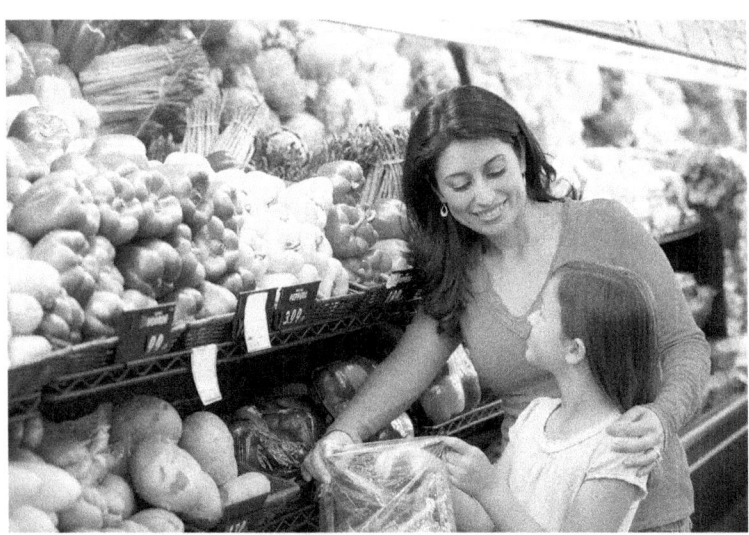

Unprocessed foods are often located in the outer perimeter of the supermarket

Fruits

All fruits are naturally gluten-free.

Eat as much as you want of unprocessed apples, apricots, avocado, bananas, cantaloupe, cherries, coconut, dates, figs, grapefruit, grapes, guava, honeydew melon, kiwi, lemon, lime, lychee, mango, oranges, papaya, peaches, pears, pineapple, plums, pomegranate, rhubarb, tangerines, watermelon, and other fruits.

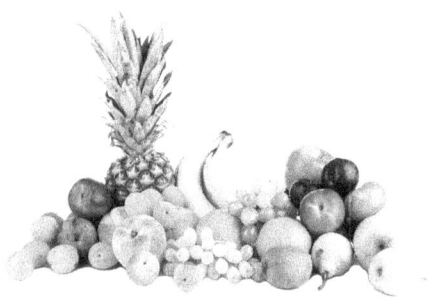

All fruits are naturally gluten-free

Berries

All berries are naturally gluten-free.

Eat your fill of unprocessed acai berries, black currants, blueberries, boysenberries, cranberries, elderberries, gooseberries, huckleberries, lingonberries, mulberries, raspberries, red currants, strawberries, and other berries.

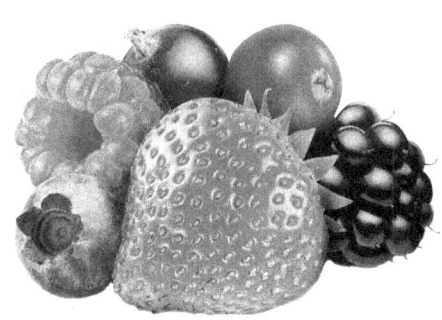

All unprocessed berries are gluten-free

Legumes

Legumes (peas, beans, and lentils) are naturally gluten-free. Common legumes include black beans, black-eyed peas, cannellini (white kidney) beans, fava beans, garbanzo beans (chickpeas), great northern beans, kidney beans, lentils, lima (butter) beans, mung beans, navy beans, peas (split peas), pinto beans, and soybeans.

Bean sprouts are also naturally gluten-free.

Most legumes are dried prior to packaging. You may safely enjoy dried legumes but examine the ingredients list before consuming legumes that have been canned, processed by methods other than drying, or packaged as a mixture of legumes and other grains (such as a soup mix that contains barley).

See the section on **Reading Food Labels** for help in determining if added ingredients are gluten-free.

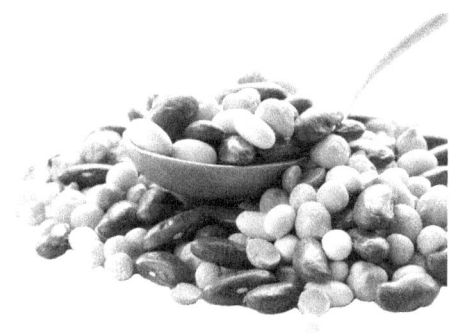

Examine the ingredients list to determine if processed legumes are gluten-free

What foods are safe to eat?

A special note about tofu

Tofu is a processed food that is made from soybeans. Because tofu is a processed food you will need to examine the ingredients list to determine if it is safe for consumption. Some tofu products are flavored with gluten-containing ingredients. A common flavoring is soy sauce which can contain wheat.

An allergy to soy products is common. Do not consume soy products if you have experienced a reaction after consuming soy.

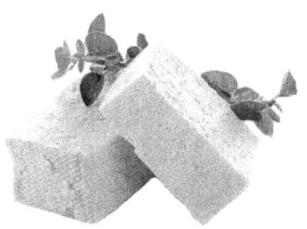

Tofu products may contain gluten

Rice

All varieties of rice are naturally gluten-free. Common types of rice include Arborio, basmati, brown rice, converted (parboiled rice), instant rice, jasmine, long grain, sticky rice, sushi rice, white rice, and wild rice.

Carefully examine the ingredients list before consuming processed rice products such as flavored rice pilafs and risotto mixes. Some flavorings and additives may contain gluten.

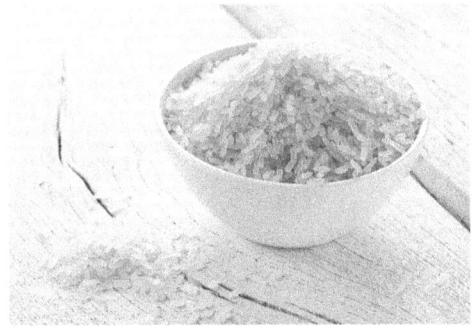

All varieties of unflavored rice are gluten-free

Corn

All varieties of corn (maize) are naturally gluten-free.

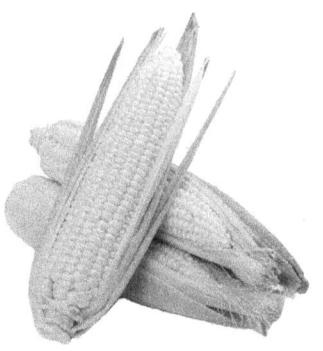

This gift from the New World to the Old World after Christopher Columbus's discovery of America meant that gluten intolerant people who couldn't eat pasta could safely enjoy polenta which is a porridge made from corn.

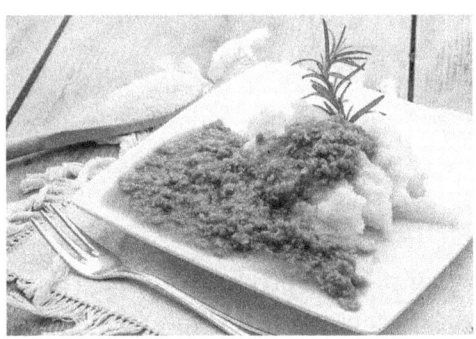

Polenta is made from ground corn and can substitute for pasta

The American version of polenta is called grits. Grits are made from hominy which consists of corn kernels that have been soaked in water and lye to remove the kernel's yellow outer hull. The hominy is then dried and ground to produce grits.

Unlike polenta which is yellow in color, grits are a creamy white color because the yellow hull has been removed prior to grinding. In Cajun and Creole cooking popular in the American South, grits are often served smothered in spicy seafood sauces (for example, Shrimp and Grits).

Those who are gluten intolerant can safely enjoy unflavored polenta, hominy, grits, corn on the cob, frozen corn kernels, and popcorn.

Carefully examine the ingredients list before consuming processed corn products such as flavored popcorn, flavored polenta, and frozen corn products that include other ingredients. Some flavorings and additives may contain gluten.

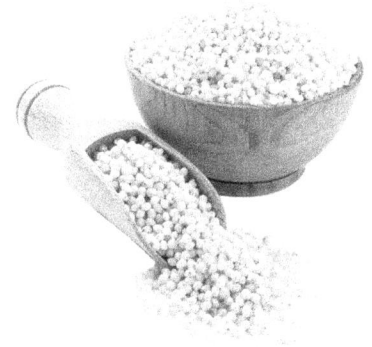

Millet can substitute for couscous in many recipes

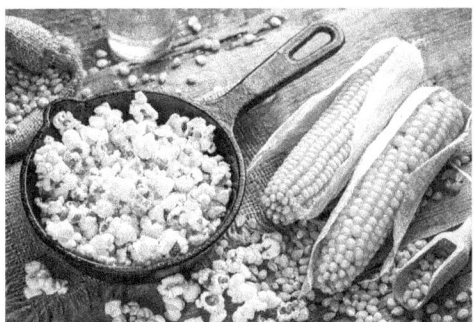

Many unprocessed (unflavored) corn products are gluten-free

Other grains

There are other less common grains that are gluten-free including millet, quinoa, amaranth, buckwheat, teff, and sorghum.

Millet is recognizable as the tiny yellow grains found in bird seed. Cooked millet looks and tastes similar to couscous but has a nuttier flavor and a chewier texture. It can substitute for couscous in many recipes.

Quinoa (pronounced "KEEN-wah") is an ancient seed that was cultivated by the Incans. Quinoa is easily digestible and is a complete protein that is superior protein-wise to wheat or rice. This makes it an excellent source of protein for vegetarians and vegans. Quinoa can be made into a pilaf or its flour can be used to make gluten-free pastas and baked goods.

Amaranth is a high-protein grain that was a staple in the diet of the ancient Aztecs but is less common today. It can be popped like popcorn. Its strong-flavored flour is sometimes used to flavor breads.

Despite its name, buckwheat is not a type of wheat but a triangular-shaped seed that is related to the rhubarb plant. It is commonly used in crepes and pancakes. It holds its shape well when cooked and can substitute for bulgur wheat or pearl barley in soups and stews.

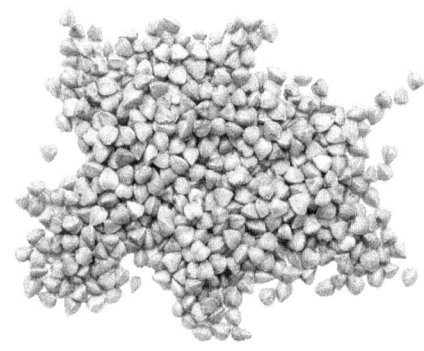

Buckwheat is gluten-free and can substitute for bulgur wheat or pearl barley

Teff is a tiny, high-protein grain that can grow in harsh climates such as those found in Ethiopia. It is used in some African countries to make flatbread. In the United States it is more commonly used to make a quick-cooking porridge that can substitute for porridges made from wheat.

Sorghum, although not a common grain in the United States, is the fifth most-cultivated cereal crop in the world after rice, wheat, corn (maize), and barley. Sorghum is extensively grown because of its high protein content, drought resistance, and ability to grow in extremes of temperature and altitude. Sorghum can be made into porridge or it can be ground into a sweet flour that is used in gluten-free baked goods.

Oats

While oats and oatmeal are naturally gluten-free they are highly susceptible to cross-contamination from other gluten-containing grains.

Oats are unsafe for those who are highly sensitive to gluten unless they have been certified as gluten-free.

See the section on **Cross Contamination** for more information on choosing oat products that are safe to consume.

Processed grains

Most rice and grains are dried prior to packaging.

Examine the ingredients list for other gluten-containing ingredients before consuming rice or other normally gluten-free grains that have been canned, were processed by methods other than drying, or have been packaged as a mixture with other grains (such as a soup mix that contains barley).

Nuts and seeds

All varieties of nuts are naturally gluten-free. Enjoy unprocessed acorns, almonds, beech nuts, Brazil nuts, cashews, chestnuts, coconuts, hazelnuts (filberts), macadamia nuts, peanuts, pecans, pine nuts, pistachios, and walnuts.

When consuming processed nuts (such as mixed nuts) check the ingredients list to ensure that no gluten-containing ingredients have been added. Occasionally manufacturers will add wheat flour as a binding agent to make flavoring adhere to the nuts.

Allergies to peanuts and tree nuts are common so do not consume nuts if you have experienced an allergic reaction after consuming them.

All varieties of edible seeds are naturally gluten-free. Enjoy unprocessed flax seeds, poppy seeds, pumpkin seeds, sesame seeds, and sunflower seeds.

Smaller seeds such as sesame seeds, flax seeds, and poppy seeds are often used in bread products and snack foods such as granola. Carefully examine the ingredients list for gluten-containing ingredients before consuming these types of foods.

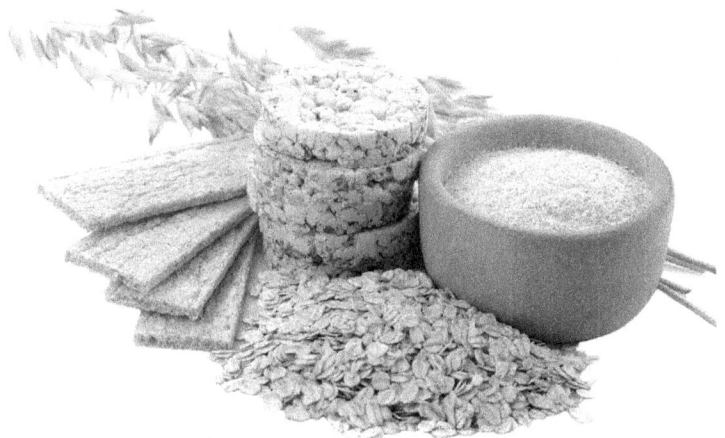

Oats are gluten-free but can easily become contaminated with gluten during processing

Sesame seed oil is also used to flavor many Asian dishes. While sesame seed allergy is not as common as allergies to peanuts or tree nuts there are a significant number of people who are allergic to sesame seeds.

Do not consume products containing sesame seeds or sesame seed oil if you have experienced a reaction to sesame seed products.

Cooking oil

Many plant-based cooking oils are made from processed nuts (coconut, palm nut, peanut, walnut), seeds (canola, cottonseed, flaxseed, safflower, sesame, sunflower), legumes (soybean), vegetables (corn), and fruits (grape seed, olive). It is not common for gluten-containing ingredients to be added to cooking oils so most cooking oils can be consumed without worry.

Do not consume cooking oils made from soybeans or sesame seeds if you have experienced an allergic reaction after consuming sesame or soy.

Mushrooms

All varieties of mushrooms are naturally gluten-free. Enjoy unprocessed commercially-available chanterelle, enokitake (enoki), oyster, porcini, portobello (crimini), shitake, and white (button) mushrooms. You may also safely enjoy truffles which are a mushroom-like fungus that grows below ground.

Mushrooms are often dried so that they can be stored without refrigeration. Before consuming dried mushrooms check the ingredients list to determine if gluten-containing ingredients have been added as anti-clumping agents or as additional flavoring.

Some wild mushrooms can be poisonous so never consume mushrooms that are harvested from the wild unless you have been properly trained in identification of poisonous mushrooms.

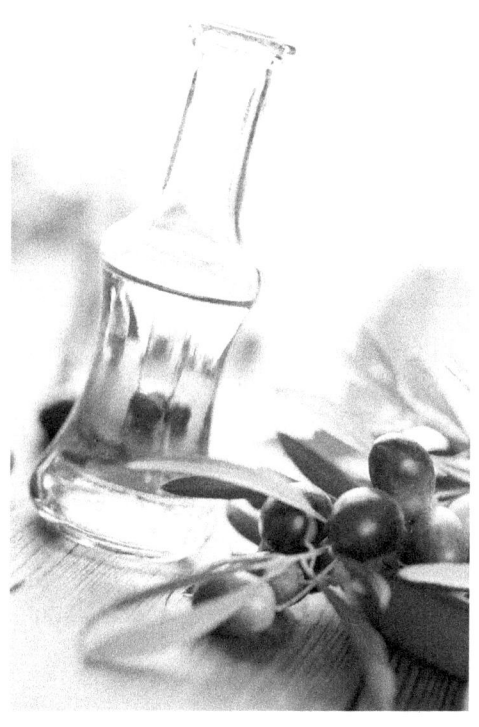

Cooking oils are gluten-free

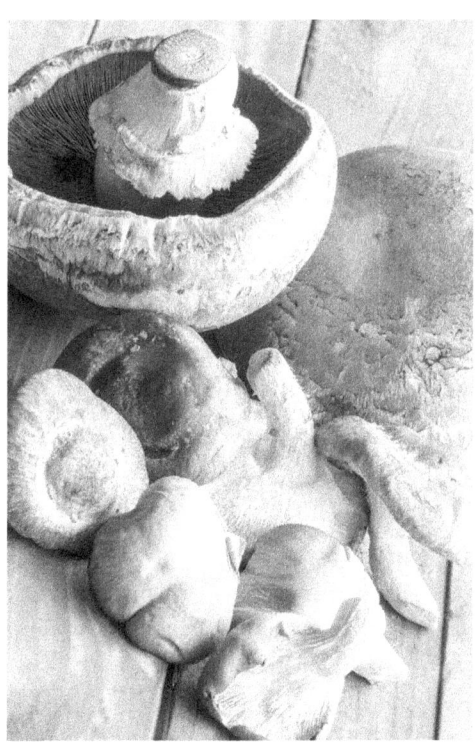

Unprocessed mushrooms are gluten-free

What foods are safe to eat?

Herbs and spices

All herbs are naturally gluten-free. Enjoy fresh or dried basil, caraway, chervil, chives, cilantro, cumin, dill, fennel, lavender, lemongrass, marjoram, mint, oregano, parsley, rosemary, sage, tarragon, and thyme.

Check the ingredients list for mixed herbal seasonings to determine if anti-caking agents that may contain gluten have been added.

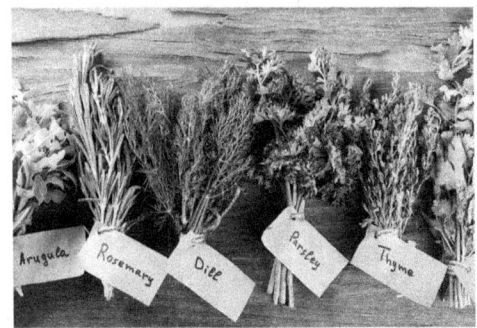

All herbs and spices are gluten-free

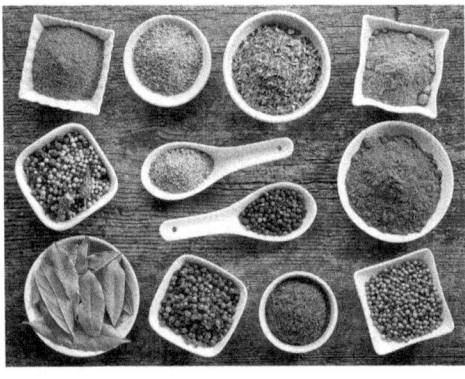

All spices are naturally gluten-free. Commercially-prepared powdered spices that contain only the named spice are generally free of cross-contamination with gluten. These spices include allspice, anise, bay leaf, cayenne pepper, chili peppers, cinnamon, cloves, coriander, ginger, juniper berry, licorice, mace, mustard, nutmeg, paprika, pepper, saffron, star anise, sumac, and turmeric.

Check the ingredients list before using commercially-prepared spice mixtures (Cajun Seasoning, Chinese Five Spice Powder, Pumpkin Pie Spice, etc.) to determine if potential gluten-containing ingredients have been added.

Dairy products

Many dairy products are naturally gluten-free

Unflavored milk (cow, sheep, goat) is gluten-free. Flavored milks (chocolate, vanilla, strawberry) may or may not contain gluten so check the ingredients list before consuming.

Processed milk products such as cream, half-and-half, crème fraîche, sour cream, ice cream, and yogurt may or may not contain gluten depending upon whether thickening agents that contain gluten were added. Consult the ingredients list carefully before consuming these processed milk products.

Many unflavored (plain) yogurts are now gluten-free. Look for the words 'gluten-free' or the letters 'GF' near the ingredients list to confirm that the yogurt is safe for consumption.

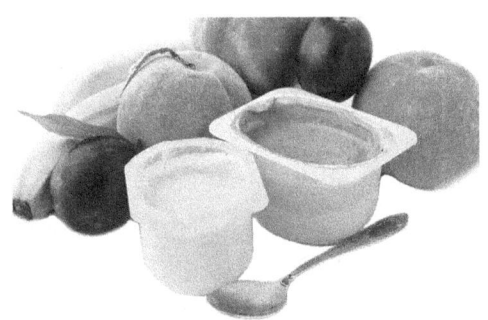

Some flavored yogurts are not gluten-free

Butter (salted, unsalted, sweet cream) is usually gluten-free.

Butter is made from the coagulated butterfat of cream. Cream is a milk product whose fat has been concentrated. Most butter is gluten-free as no gluten-containing additives are necessary to coagulate the butterfat into a solid.

Margarine is an emulsion of vegetable oil and water that may or may not contain milk products. Vegans who wish to avoid animal products or those who need to avoid animal fat for health reasons may need to substitute a vegetable-based margarine for butter.

Vegetable oils do not easily coagulate into a solid so many margarines contain additives to thicken and solidify the oils and to add color and flavor. These additives may contain gluten. When using margarine select a brand that is labeled 'gluten-free'.

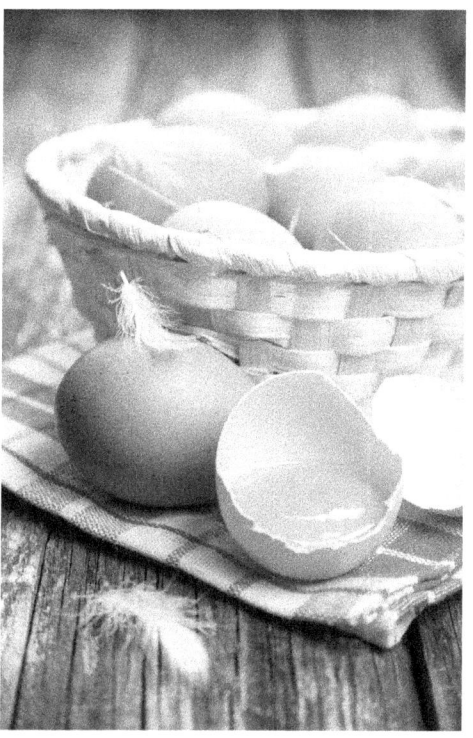

*Butter is usually gluten-free
Margarine may contain gluten*

Unprocessed eggs (in the shell) are naturally gluten-free. Enjoy unprocessed chicken, duck, goose, quail, and other wild and domestic eggs.

Processed egg products such as pre-shelled, pre-beaten egg mixtures may or may not contain gluten. Many of these products contain colorings and flavorings. Consult the ingredients list before consuming.

*Unprocessed eggs in the shell
are gluten-free*

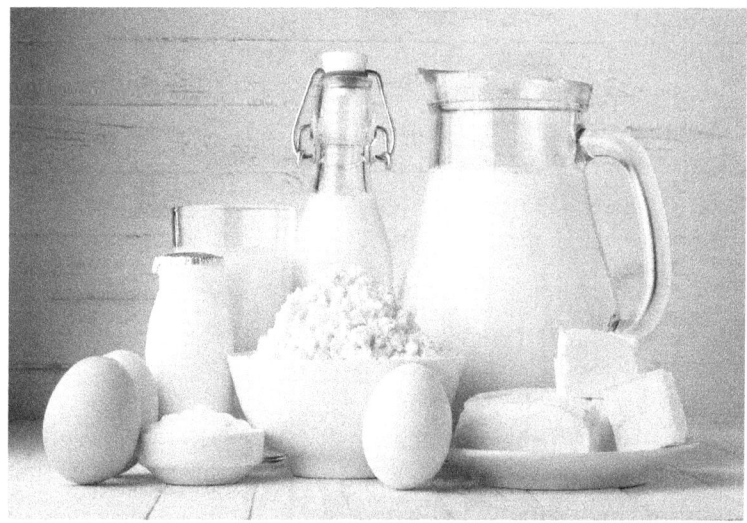

Many dairy products are naturally gluten-free

What foods are safe to eat? 23

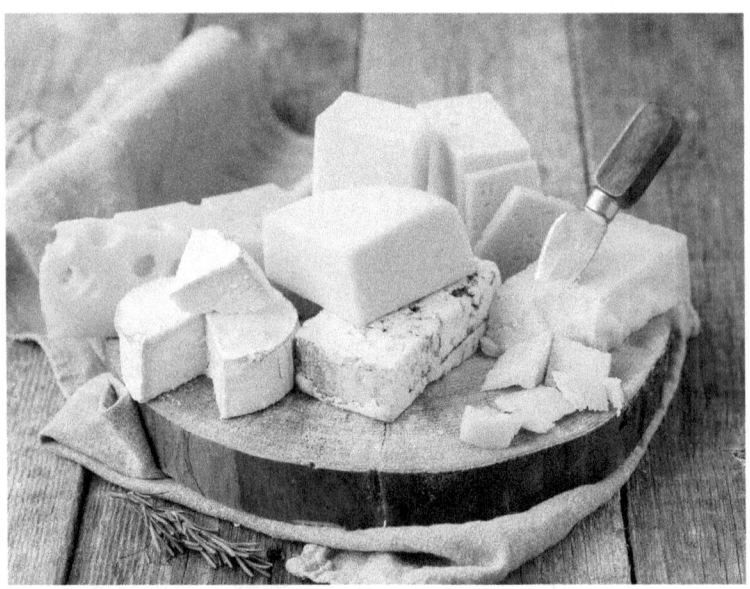

*Many types of cheese do not contain gluten
Blue cheese may contain gluten*

A special note about cheese

Many types of cheese are gluten-free. Commonly available bulk cheeses such as Cheddar, Swiss, Mozzarella, Parmesan, Colby, and Monterey Jack rarely contain gluten. These cheeses are safe to consume as long as they have not been grated or shredded.

Be cautious when using grated or shredded cheeses. Anti-clumping agents added to cheese after grating or shredding may contain gluten so check the ingredients list carefully. When in doubt, buy bulk cheese and grate or shred it yourself. More manufacturers are using cellulose (made from wood) or corn-based starches as anti-clumping agents instead of gluten-containing starches which were used in the past.

Some brands of soft cheeses such as cottage cheese and ricotta can contain gluten which helps to thicken them. Some processed cheeses such as spreadable cheese, loaf and jar cheeses, and processed cheese slices may also contain gluten as a thickening agent. Inspect the ingredients list for gluten-containing ingredients before consuming processed cheese or soft cheeses.

All beer-washed cheeses will likely contain gluten so avoid beer-washed cheeses.

Blue cheese

Use extra caution when consuming blue cheeses which can contain gluten. Stilton, Roquefort, Limburger, Gorgonzola and other types of blue cheeses are made by injecting the cheese with a bacterial culture (commonly Penicillium Roqueforti) that causes the blue and blue-green pockets and veins in the cheese.

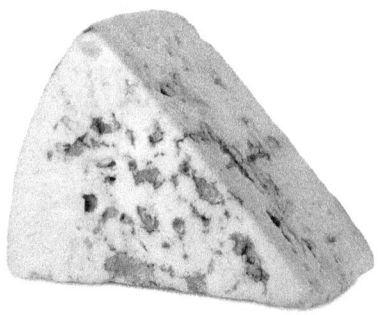

*Some types of blue cheese
are not gluten-free*

The bacterial culture is often grown on bread crumbs or the grains or malts of wheat and rye, all of which contain gluten. To further complicate matters, unless the cheese is specifically marked gluten-free it is difficult to determine whether the bacterial culture was grown on a medium that contained gluten.

If the bacterial culture that was used was grown on a medium that contained gluten then the cheese may contain a very small amount of gluten. Some people have found they can tolerate this extremely small amount of gluten. If you are highly sensitive to gluten then avoid blue cheese or purchase a blue cheese labeled 'gluten-free'.

Meats

All unprocessed meats (beef, pork, lamb, buffalo, venison, wild game) are naturally gluten-free. Unprocessed meats are those that haven't been cured, dried, brined, marinated, breaded, or injected with a flavoring solution.

Enjoy unprocessed meats such as beef steak, pork chops, hamburger, lamb, veal, venison, rabbit, and other wild game. You may add gluten-free herbs, spices, and marinades during cooking or grilling.

Use caution when consuming processed meats such as ham, bacon, Canadian bacon, sausage, chorizo, jerky, pepperoni, salami, and other meat products made with additives. Examine the ingredients list carefully for gluten. See the section on **Reading Food Labels** for help in determining if a processed meat contains gluten.

Poultry

All unprocessed poultry is naturally gluten-free. Unprocessed poultry is poultry that hasn't been breaded, brined, marinated, or injected with a flavoring solution. This includes unprocessed chicken, turkey, duck, goose, Cornish game hen, quail, pheasant, and other types of domesticated and wild poultry.

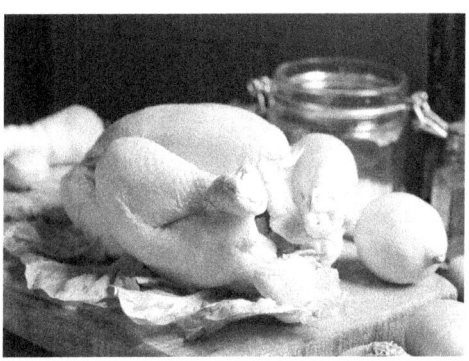

Unprocessed poultry is gluten-free

Use caution when consuming processed turkeys that may have been injected with a flavoring solution containing wheat starch.

Be sure to carefully inspect the ingredients list when using ground turkey and ground chicken because these processed poultry products often contain additives which may not be gluten-free.

See the section on **Reading Food Labels** for help in identifying whether processed poultry products are gluten-free.

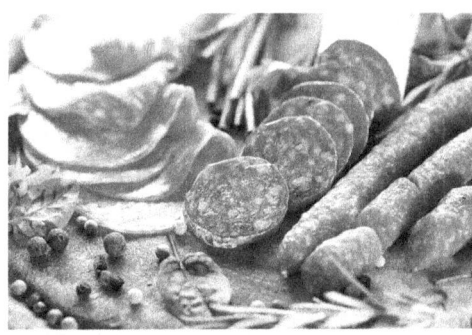
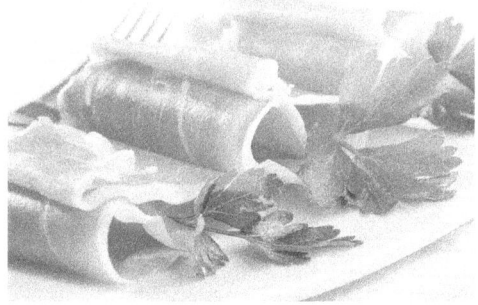

Processed meats may contain gluten

Fish

All unprocessed fish (saltwater, freshwater) and all unprocessed eels are naturally gluten-free. Unprocessed fish products are those that haven't been marinated, battered, breaded, frozen with additives, dried, smoked, canned in broth, or tinned in oil.

Enjoy unprocessed anchovy, cod, catfish, eel, flounder, grouper, haddock, hake, halibut, herring, mackerel, mahi mahi, monkfish, mullet, orange roughy, pike, pollock, salmon, sardines, sea bass, shark, snapper, sole, sturgeon, swordfish, tilapia, trout, tuna, turbot, wahoo, and whitefish.

Use caution when consuming processed fish products. Marinated fish products may contain soy sauce which often contains small amounts of wheat. See the section on **Reading Food Labels** for help in identifying whether a processed fish product is gluten-free.

Canned or tinned fish may contain gluten. In the past many manufacturers of water-packed tuna flavored their products with a broth that contained wheat. Because of the increasing awareness of gluten sensitivity it is becoming more common for canned tuna to be flavored with vegetable broths (usually soy flavoring). Some manufacturers have eliminated the flavorings and are packing their tuna in a salt and water brine.

Most fish packed in oil does not intentionally contain gluten. This includes oil-packed tuna, sardines, and kippers. Check the ingredients list for gluten-containing additives before consuming oil-packed fish.

When possible select a tuna that has been labeled gluten-free. If you are unable to find gluten-free tuna packed in a water broth you can substitute oil-packed tuna. Drain the oil-packed tuna in a metal sieve. Rinse the fish gently with a hot water spray to remove the oil. Allow the excess water to drain before using.

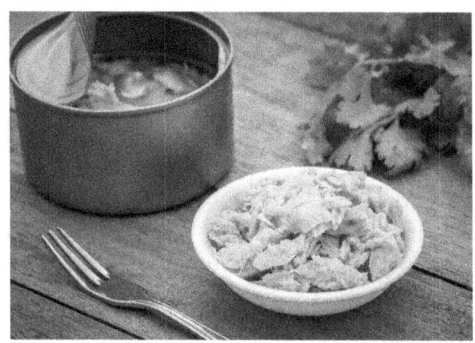

Some canned tunas contain gluten

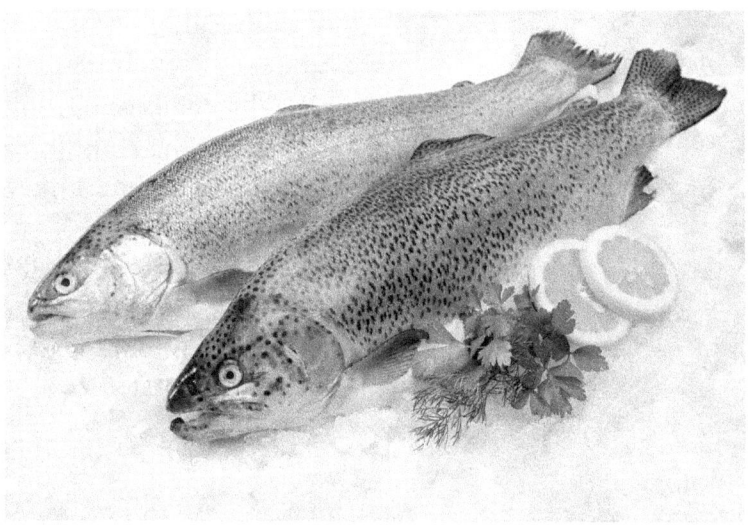

Unprocessed fish is gluten-free

Shellfish

All unprocessed shellfish (saltwater, freshwater) is naturally gluten-free as are unprocessed mollusks such as octopus, cuttlefish, and squid. Unprocessed shellfish is shellfish whose shell has not been removed and whose flesh has not been marinated, battered, breaded, brined, frozen with additives, dried, smoked, canned in broth, tinned in oil, or injected with a flavoring solution.

You may safely eat unprocessed abalone, anemone, clams, conch, crab, crawfish, crayfish, cuttlefish, langoustines, lobster, mussels, octopus, oysters, prawns, scallops, sea cucumber, sea urchin, shrimp, squid, and whelk.

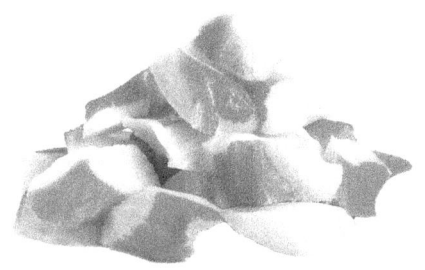

Imitation crab meat often contains gluten

Use extra caution when consuming processed crabmeat, especially products labeled 'imitation crabmeat' which may also be labeled as 'surimi'. Most brands of imitation crabmeat are made from a mixture of ground fish that often includes wheat as an ingredient.

Shellfish allergies are common. Do not consume shellfish products if you have had an allergic reaction to shellfish in the past.

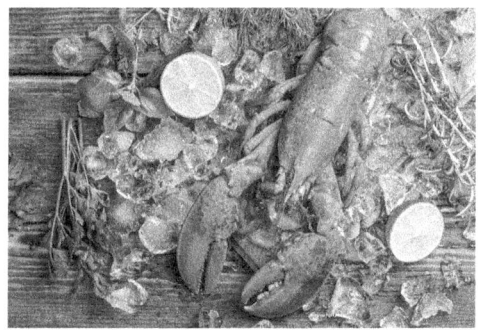

Unprocessed shellfish is gluten-free

Use caution when consuming processed shellfish and mollusks. Check the ingredients list carefully for additives such as flavorings and brines that may contain gluten. Marinated shellfish products may contain soy sauce which often contains small amounts of wheat. See the section on **Reading Food Labels** for help in identifying whether a processed shellfish product is gluten-free.

Wine

All unfortified wines are naturally gluten-free. Wine is made from the juice of red or white grapes which is fermented with yeast to convert the sugar in the grapes into alcohol. Unfortified wines do not contain additives that contain gluten.

Fortified wines are wines that have distilled spirits (such as brandy) added to them. Some distilled spirits contain Caramel Coloring which is often made from wheat so fortified wines are generally not safe to consume.

Fortified wines including port, sherry, Madeira, Masala, and vermouth should be avoided unless they are specifically labeled 'gluten-free'.

Use caution when consuming wine coolers as some wine coolers are flavored with ingredients that contain gluten.

What foods are safe to eat?

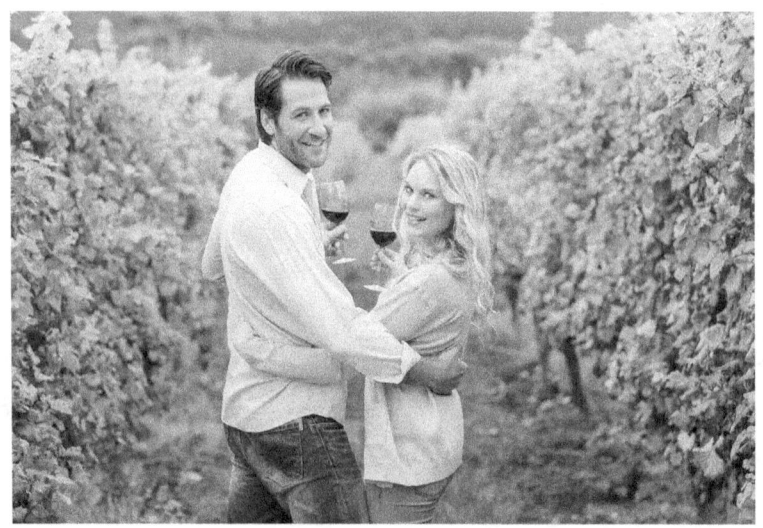

Unfortified wines are gluten-free

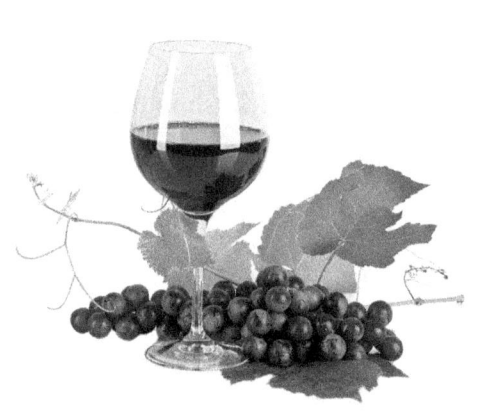

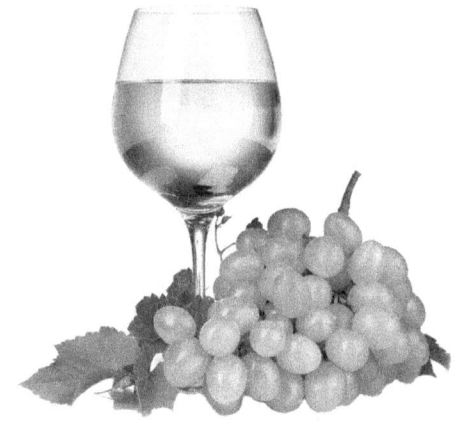

Enjoy unfortified red wines such as Barbera, Cabernet Franc, Cabernet Sauvignon, Grenache, Malbec, Merlot, Petit Verdot, Pinot Noir, Sangiovese, Syrah, Zinfandel, and blends of these varietals.

Enjoy unfortified white wines such as Chardonnay, Pinot Blanc, Pinot Grigio, Riesling, Rosé, Sauvignon Blanc, and blends of these varietals.

Sparkling white wines such as Champagne are also safe for consumption.

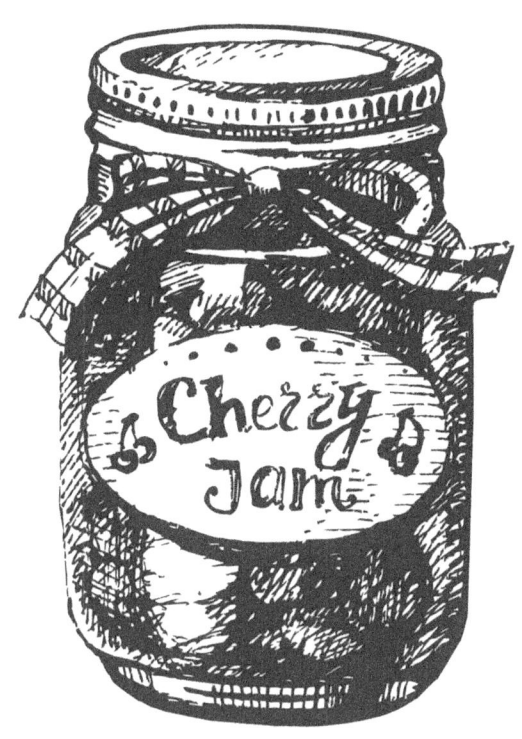

Reading Food Labels

Major food allergens

In 2004 the United States Food and Drug Administration (USFDA) Food Allergen Labeling and Consumer Protection Act mandated that food ingredient labels must call out 'major food allergens'.

This labeling rule applies to food products manufactured in the USA and certain imported foods that are subject to USFDA regulation.

The major food allergens are currently defined as follows: milk, eggs, fish, shellfish, tree nuts, peanuts, wheat, and soybeans. These eight major allergens account for over ninety percent of documented food allergies.

It is important to note that gluten intolerance is not a food allergy per se and does not typically result in the immediate life-threatening symptoms associated with food allergies such as anaphylaxis (swelling, hives, and dangerously low blood pressure).

However, those who are gluten intolerant have benefitted greatly from the USFDA rules because they require that all food products that contain wheat clearly state this information on the label. Wheat is the primary source of gluten in the American diet, with products containing barley and rye being a much smaller proportion.

What this means is that it is now much easier to identify whether a processed or packaged food contains gluten.

How do I read a food label?

Products manufactured in the United States that contain wheat as an ingredient will list that information on the product's ingredient label in one or both of the following ways:

The label will use the word "CONTAINS" followed closely by the word "WHEAT".

In the "INGREDIENTS" list the name of the 'food source' will follow the ingredient and will be contained in parenthesis ( ).

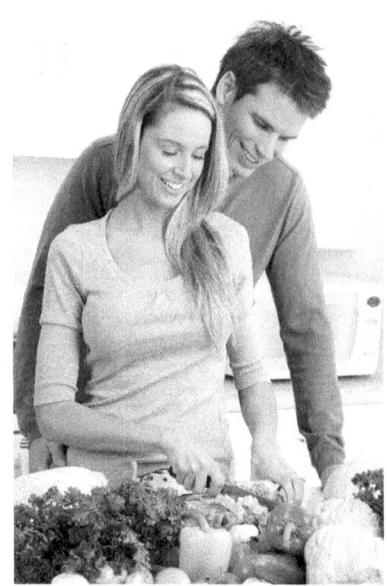

Learning to identify what foods contain gluten makes cooking gluten-free easy

All food sources that indicate the words "WHEAT", "BARLEY", or "RYE" are not safe for consumption by those who are gluten intolerant.

The food label given in the example below indicates that the product is not gluten-free for the following reasons:

The allergen information states that the product

CONTAINS: WHEAT

The food source for the ingredient listed as

ENRICHED FLOUR is WHEAT FLOUR.

The ingredient listing contains

MALTED BARLEY FLOUR.

The ingredient listing contains

CARAMEL COLOR

which is often made from wheat. See the section on **Food Additives** for more information.

It is important to note that BARLEY and RYE are not considered major food allergens so they will not be called out in the allergen information given after the word 'CONTAINS'. You must inspect the INGREDIENTS listing to check for them there.

INGREDIENTS: ENRICHED FLOUR (WHEAT FLOUR, NIACIN, THIAMINE), SOY FLOUR, SUGAR, HYDROGENATED COCONUT OIL, MOLASSES, CORNSTARCH, MALTED BARLEY FLOUR, CARAMEL COLOR, SALT

CONTAINS: WHEAT, SOY

MANUFACTURED ON EQUIPMENT THAT PROCESSES: PEANUTS, MILK

An ingredient label for a product that is not gluten-free

Cross-contamination

Cross-contamination is the unintentional contamination of a normally gluten-free product with small amounts of gluten that have been introduced during manufacturing of the product.

While not required by the USFDA many food labels give information on cross-contamination. Labeling information on cross-contamination typically includes the words "MANUFACTURED ON EQUIPMENT THAT PROCESSES WHEAT".

Cross-contamination information will only address the eight major allergens which include WHEAT. Cross-contamination with barley and rye will not be called out.

This means that if all the ingredients in a product are gluten-free, all the food sources are gluten-free, wheat is not listed as an allergen, and the product was not manufactured on equipment that processes wheat you can still experience a reaction if your food was cross-contaminated with barley or rye. Fortunately, cross-contamination with barley or rye is uncommon.

Many people who are not extremely sensitive to gluten will assume the risk and consume a product that lists WHEAT as a possible cross-contaminant as long as the product does not intentionally contain wheat, barley, and rye (as indicated by the ingredients listing and allergen information). As always, if consuming a food causes symptoms do not continue to consume that food.

In addition to the potential for cross-contamination during manufacturing, food can also be contaminated with gluten during food preparation in the home or at a restaurant. See the section on *Cookware and Utensils* for tips on avoiding cross-contamination during food preparation.

Oats are gluten-free - why do I get a reaction when I eat them?

Oats are the food source for oatmeal and oat flour which is an ingredient in many breakfast cereals and breads. Oats are naturally gluten-free but they physically resemble other gluten-containing grains in both size and shape, making them highly susceptible to cross-contamination.

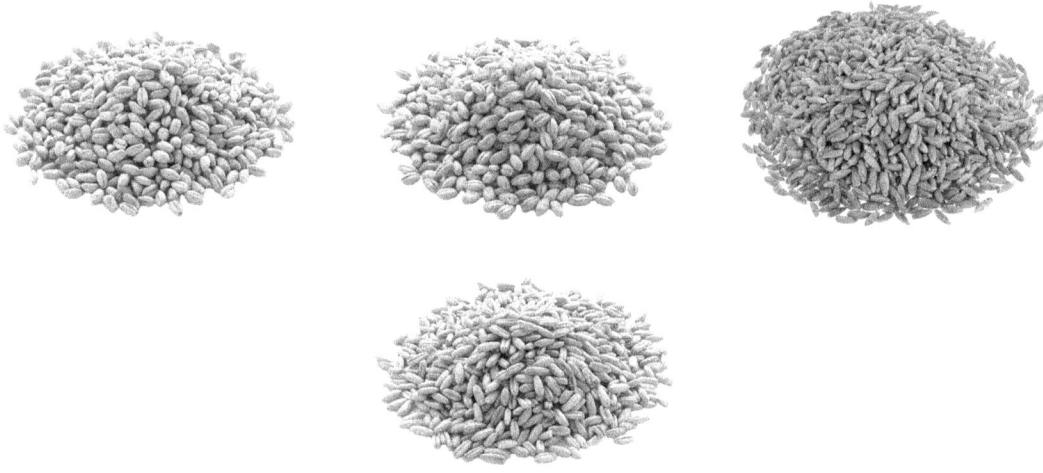

Top row: wheat, barley, and rye
Bottom row: oats

Reading Food Labels

Cross-contamination can occur during:

Growing of Crops

Stray wheat, barley, or rye seeds can germinate in an oat field. All four grains can be grown in the same field on alternating years (crop rotation) and are often harvested, shipped, and milled using the same equipment. This makes the potential for cross-contamination very high.

Harvest and Shipping

Oats are harvested by farm equipment that previously harvested wheat, barley, or rye and/or the oats were shipped in a truck that previously contained wheat, barley, or rye. Unless the harvesting and shipping equipment is meticulously cleaned cross-contamination can occur.

Milling and Manufacturing

Rollers, grindstones, and conveyer belts can retain trace amounts of the flours from wheat, barley, or rye that can contaminate oats that are processed on the same equipment.

Wheat, barley, and rye grains are similar in size and shape to oat grains, making it difficult to use screening methods to separate them during manufacturing.

Should I buy gluten-free oatmeal?

Because gluten-free oat grains are so similar in size and shape to their gluten-containing cousins (wheat, barley, and rye) it is difficult to avoid cross-contamination. For a manufacturer to certify their oat-containing products as gluten-free they must go to great lengths to regulate their oat suppliers and their milling processes.

Many manufacturers of gluten-free products also test their finished product for gluten as part of their quality control process. This is why oatmeal that is certified 'gluten-free' is more expensive than regular oatmeal.

For those who are extremely sensitive to gluten it is best to buy oatmeal that is certified 'gluten-free'. For those who are not highly sensitive and wish to reduce costs then the consumption of regular oatmeal may be an option.

If consuming 'regular' oatmeal causes symptoms do not continue to consume it. Purchase oatmeal that is certified 'gluten-free'.

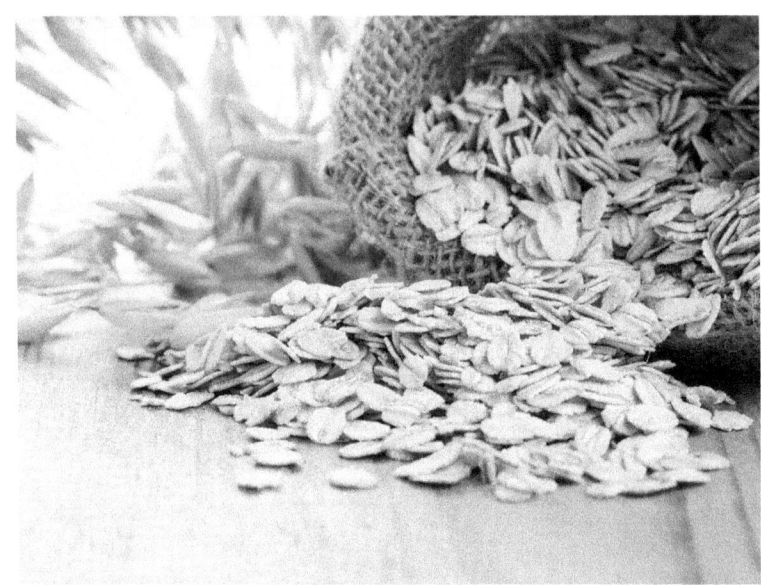

Certified gluten-free oatmeal is worth the extra expense

Is it safe to eat rice and corn?

Rice and corn are both naturally gluten-free. Rice and corn, along with beans and other legumes, form the carbohydrate staples of the western gluten-free diet. Many people who are gluten intolerant are able to eat 'regular' rice and corn that have not been certified as gluten-free without experiencing symptoms. This is because rice and corn are less susceptible to cross-contamination.

Rice and corn kernels have significantly different shapes that make them easier to differentiate from wheat, barley, and rye grains which are small and somewhat spherical. Rice is an elongated grain with a husk and corn is a large grain that has a boxy shape.

There are also big differences in the way rice and corn are grown and harvested as compared to cultivation of wheat, barley, and rye.

Rice is usually grown in fields that are flooded for part of the growing cycle (rice paddies). Crop rotation with wheat, barley, and rye is rare. In addition, rice is harvested using machinery that is significantly different from the machinery used to harvest wheat, barley, and rye.

These different cultivation and harvesting techniques make cross-contamination of rice with wheat, barley, and rye far less likely.

Corn is often grown in fields where wheat, barley, and rye have been grown but cross-contamination is not as likely because corn kernels are still attached to a large cob during the first stages of harvesting. The machinery that separates the cob from the cornstalk is sized to prefer the collection of the large corn cob versus the small ear of wheat, barley, or rye which typically falls to the ground during collection of the cob.

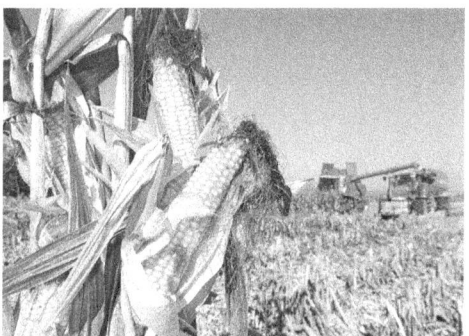

Corn kernels are attached to their cob during the first stage of harvesting

After the corn kernels have been separated from the cob it is relatively easy to differentiate them from gluten-containing grains. Corn kernels are significantly larger and heavier than grains of wheat, barley, or rye. This makes it easier for gravity and screening processes to separate out the larger, heavier gluten-free corn kernels from any smaller, lighter gluten-containing grains that may contaminate them.

For this reason, most people who are gluten intolerant do not experience symptoms when they consume 'regular' rice and corn that has not been certified as 'gluten-free'.

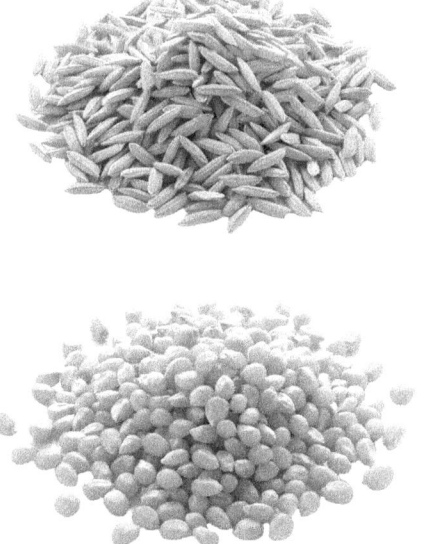

Top: Rice (with husk intact)
Bottom: Corn

Products labeled 'gluten-free'

In 2013 the USFDA established a threshold by which a food can be labeled 'gluten-free'. The labeling of a product as 'gluten-free' is currently voluntary by the manufacturer. Given the premium pricing that manufacturers can charge for products that are labeled gluten-free it benefits them to label qualifying products as such.

The USFDA does not specify how the manufacturer must label gluten-free products but in general, a product that falls within the USFDA guidelines for being gluten-free will be marked in one or more of the following ways:

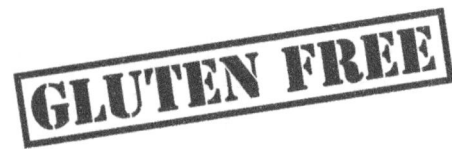

*With the words
'Gluten Free' or 'Gluten-Free'*

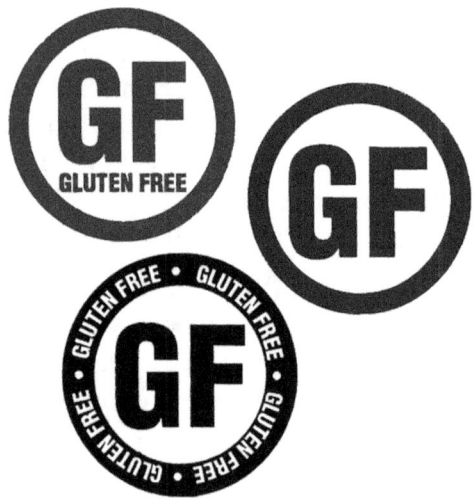

With the letters 'GF'

How do you define 'gluten-free'?

The threshold for a product to be considered gluten-free has been defined by the USFDA to be under 20 parts per million (ppm) of gluten. 20 ppm is equivalent to 20 milligrams (20 mg) of gluten per 1 kilogram (1,000 g) of food.

For many, this threshold is adequate to avoid symptoms of gluten intolerance. For those who are extremely sensitive, products that contain amounts of gluten that are near the upper limit of the threshold may cause reactions. As with any food product you consume, if consumption causes symptoms do not continue to consume the food.

One caveat to be aware of: the current rules do not require the manufacturer to test for presence of gluten in finished food products. Some manufacturers who have forgone testing have been called on the carpet when gluten has inadvertently entered their manufacturing process.

Per the USFDA, manufacturers do bear the responsibility (and are subject to regulatory action) if gluten is found in products that they have labeled as gluten-free. Most manufacturers are conscientious about adhering to the rules as the gluten-free community has a large on-line presence and is very vocal about calling out manufacturers who fail to self-monitor for presence of gluten in their products.

What about food additives?

The list of all food additives is too large to reproduce here. The following is a list of common food additives:

Safe food additives

Guar Gum – guar gum is used as a food thickening agent because it is effective in much smaller quantities than other thickeners such as cornstarch. It is also found in some pharmaceutical drugs and cosmetics. Guar gum is made from guar seeds which are naturally gluten-free. Avoid if you are allergic to soy as the manufacturing process used to create guar gum can add soy protein impurities.

Xanthan Gum – xanthan gum is commonly used as a food thickening agent and is responsible for the spongy 'spring' in gluten-free baked goods. It is usually made from the excess whey (milk) left over during cheese production. Avoid if you have a milk allergy or must avoid casein (a milk protein) in your diet.

Cellulose – cellulose is derived from plant fibers, mainly wood pulp and cotton. Powdered cellulose is often added to shredded or grated cheeses as an anti-clumping agent.

Annatto Coloring – annatto coloring is an orange-red food coloring made from the seeds of the achiote tree. Its most common use is for adding color to Cheddar cheese and margarine. A small number of people have experienced an allergic reaction to this common food additive. Avoid if you have experienced a reaction after eating foods that contain this additive.

Gelatin – gelatin is used as a gelling agent in food, pharmaceutical drugs, and some cosmetics. It is made from the skin, bones, and connective tissues of cattle, poultry, and fish and is naturally gluten-free. Avoid if you do not consume animal products for philosophical reasons or wish to adhere to a vegan diet.

Safe when manufactured in USA

The following food additives are gluten-free when used in products manufactured in the USA.

Starch – if the product is manufactured in the USA then 'starch' is always made from corn unless the food source lists otherwise. Corn is naturally gluten-free. Avoid products that list 'starch' as an ingredient if the product is manufactured outside the USA and the food source is not given.

Maltodextrin – if the product is manufactured in the USA then 'maltodextrin' is made from corn, potatoes, or rice which are all naturally gluten-free. Avoid products that list 'maltodextrin' as the ingredient if the product is manufactured outside the USA and the food source is not given.

Modified Food Starch – if the product is manufactured in the USA then 'modified food starch' is commonly made from corn, tapioca, or potatoes which are all naturally gluten-free. If the food source is wheat then this must be listed in the allergen information and the product must be avoided. Avoid 'modified food starch' if the product is manufactured outside the USA and the food source is not given.

Hydrolyzed Whey Protein – the food source for 'hydrolyzed whey protein' is milk which is naturally gluten-free. Avoid products that contain 'hydrolyzed whey protein' if you have a milk allergy or you must avoid casein (a milk protein) in your diet.

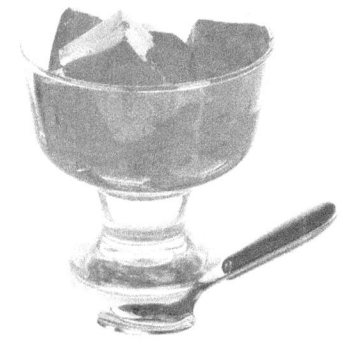

Gelatin is a gluten-free food additive

Questionable food additives

The following food additives often cause reactions for those who are gluten intolerant:

Monosodium Glutamate (MSG)

Monosodium glutamate is commonly made from sugar beets, sugar cane, molasses, and tapioca which are naturally gluten-free. Many people who are gluten intolerant are sensitive to this additive. Avoid if you are sensitive or observe symptoms of headache, numbness, or heart palpitations after consuming.

Hydrolyzed Vegetable Protein (HVP) or Hydrolyzed Plant Protein (HPP)

Commonly found in sausages, hot dogs, and meat replacements ('mock meats'), these proteins can be made from soy, corn, rice and wheat. Avoid if the food source is not identified or if the food source is soy and you have an allergy to soy products.

Yeast Extract /Autolyzed Yeast Extract

Yeast are single-celled microorganisms responsible for rising bread dough and fermenting the ingredients in wine and beer into alcohol.

Yeast extracts are made by breaking down the yeast cell wall and extracting the interior contents of the yeast cell.

Autolyzed yeast and its extracts are made from yeast cells that are allowed to die to allow the yeast proteins to break down.

Yeast extract and autolyzed yeast extract are used to impart a savory flavor in foods. It is common for manufacturers to use them as a substitute for monosodium glutamate (MSG).

Like MSG, some people also report reactions after eating products that contain yeast extracts. Avoid yeast extracts if you have a yeast allergy or observe symptoms after consuming these food additives.

Unsafe food additives

Carmel Color – avoid unless the product is specifically labeled 'gluten-free'. Caramel color can be made from wheat, barley, and their malts.

Malt or Malt Flavoring – avoid unless the food source is given and is not wheat, barley, or rye. Barley malt is the most common malt used as a flavoring but occasionally corn (which is gluten-free) is used to produce the malt.

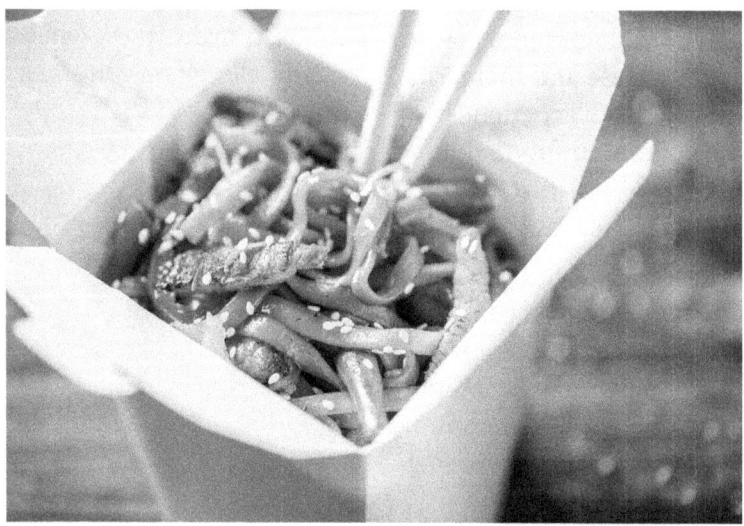

MSG is an ingredient in many Asian foods

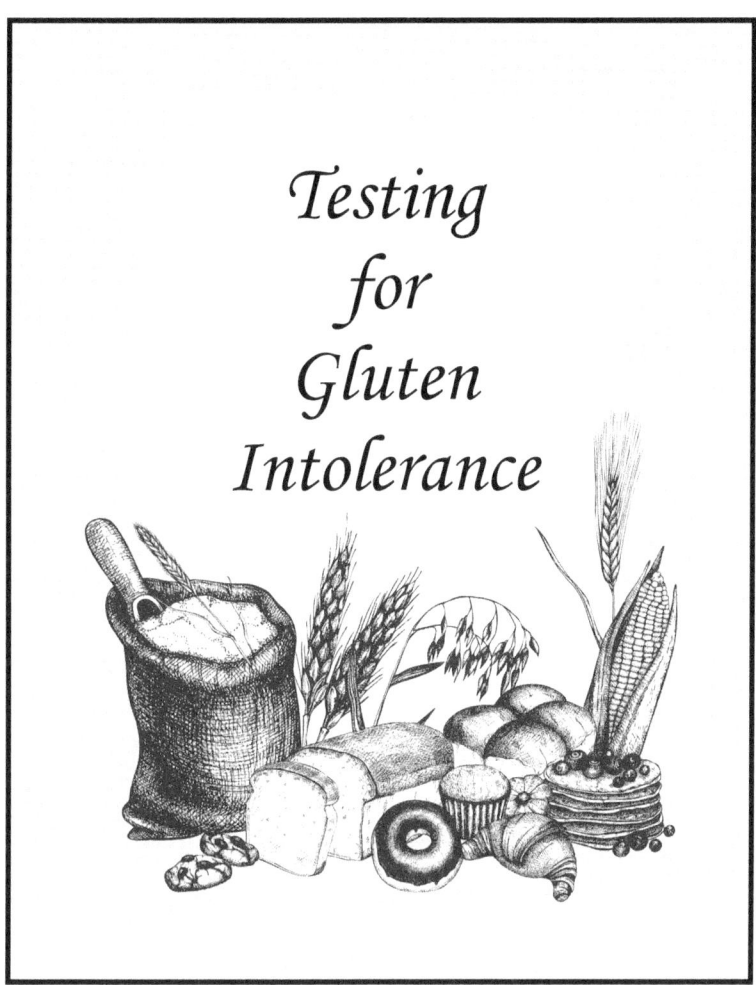

Testing for Gluten Intolerance

Why test for gluten intolerance?

Making the choice to remove gluten from your diet requires some deliberation and often requires input from your doctor.

While there are no adverse side effects to removing gluten from your diet it should be acknowledged that making the decision to go gluten-free is not an easy commitment. Gluten is found in many processed foods due to the high prevalence of wheat flour in the modern diet.

As a comparison, choosing to give up smoking requires you to abstain from cigarettes and pipe tobacco. Choosing to become a vegan requires you to forego foods made with animal products. In both these cases the products you need to avoid are usually easily identifiable.

Not so with gluten. Gluten lurks in the most unlikely of foods. For example, imitation crab meat is often made with gluten-containing wheat flour, rum can be colored with Caramel Color (often made from wheat), and even the seemingly innocuous act of drinking a beer (made with barley) can give you a dose of gluten.

Gluten can lurk in vitamins, lipstick, and places you'd never dream of looking - like the glue used to seal an envelope.

Therefore, before making the commitment to go gluten-free, many people believe that it is important to make an informed decision that includes gluten intolerance testing.

That being said, some people make the decision to go gluten-free 'cold turkey' without input from their doctor.

As mentioned previously, there are no adverse side effects that can occur after adopting a gluten-free diet without seeking input from your doctor. There is, however, a danger with regards to misdiagnosis of your symptoms.

Serious conditions such as Cystic Fibrosis and parasitic infections of the intestines can mimic the symptoms of gluten intolerance.

Only a medical professional can evaluate whether your symptoms are due to gluten intolerance or another health condition that mimics the symptoms of gluten intolerance.

Going gluten-free without input from your doctor can possibly delay treatment of a serious medical problem that is masquerading as gluten intolerance.

For this reason, many people choose to test for gluten intolerance before going gluten-free.

Whatever your decision, keep your doctor informed of your symptoms and your choice to adopt the gluten-free diet.

Methods of testing

There are a number of different methods which can be used to test for gluten intolerance. The most common methods of testing, categorized from most invasive to least invasive, are as follows:

Endoscopy with Intestinal Biopsy

Endoscopy is an invasive method of testing for intestinal damage caused by gluten intolerance. The endoscopy must be performed in a doctor's office and requires the patient to be sedated or put under anesthesia during the procedure.

During the procedure the doctor will insert a thin, flexible endoscope with a lighted camera into the patient's small intestine to determine if damage to the intestine has occurred. While the endoscope is inserted, a biopsy (tissue sample) will usually be taken. This tissue sample can be further studied under a microscope to determine the extent to which the patient's intestinal lining is damaged.

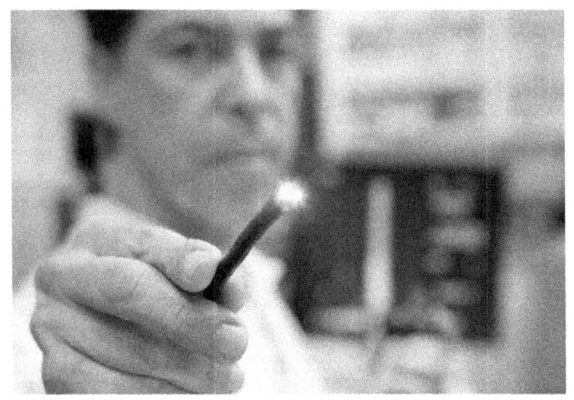

An endoscope can be used to examine the small intestine for damage

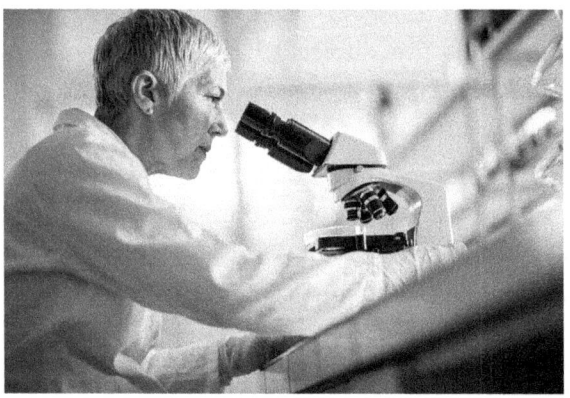

A tissue sample taken during endoscopy can be examined for intestinal damage

Endoscopy with intestinal biopsy is a highly conclusive method of testing for those whose gluten intolerance has progressed to intestinal damage. It is not necessarily conclusive for young patients with mild gluten intolerance and strong bodies that repair intestinal damage quickly. It is possible to be gluten intolerant and not have noticeable intestinal damage (no positive diagnosis of Celiac Disease).

Celiac Disease, which is the result of prolonged ingestion of gluten, is confirmed by presence of intestinal damage which is usually discovered by endoscopy. Therefore, endoscopy is the primary method of obtaining a conclusive diagnosis of Celiac Disease.

The disadvantage of endoscopy testing is that it is invasive, must be performed in a doctor's office, and is expensive if you don't have insurance; although most insurance covers this diagnostic test.

The advantage to undergoing endoscopy to obtain a formal diagnosis of Celiac Disease is that in the United States, school-aged children (including students enrolled in college) who have been diagnosed with Celiac Disease are covered under the Americans with Disabilities Act (ADA).

What this means is that your child's school or college is required by law to accommodate their special diet by offering at least one gluten-free menu choice or a gluten-free meal prepared specially for them.

Because the benefit of being eligible to receive a gluten-free meal is very desirable many parents opt to test their children via endoscopy, despite the fact that this test is invasive.

It should be noted that although schools are not required by law to provide gluten-free meals to students who are gluten intolerant but have not yet been diagnosed with Celiac Disease, some schools are offering the benefit of a gluten-free meal to non-diagnosed students who request it.

Parents of school-aged children may want to ask their school if a gluten-free meal is available without the formal diagnosis of Celiac Disease.

Adults who suspect they are gluten intolerant should consult with their doctor to determine if there is a need to undergo endoscopy to determine the extent of possible intestinal damage.

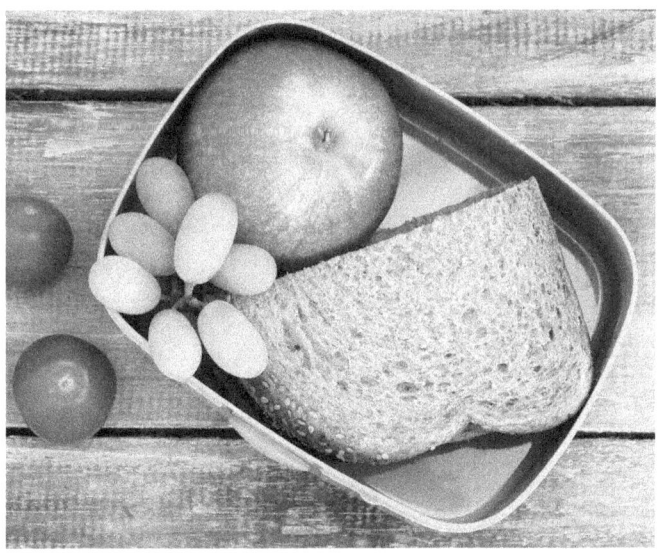

School children in America who are diagnosed with Celiac Disease are eligible for a gluten-free lunch

Antibody Blood Tests

A less invasive method of testing for gluten intolerance involves taking a sample of the patient's blood and testing for antibodies that are produced when the patient's body reacts to gluten.

Many doctors use the Tissue Transglutaminase Antibodies (tTG-IgA) test as a starting point to check for gluten intolerance. Note that this test must be performed prior to the start of a gluten-free diet as the test checks for antibodies that are generated in response to the patient's ingestion of gluten.

The tTG-IgA test will be positive for approximately 98% of patients with Celiac Disease who have eaten gluten-containing foods prior to testing. Because this test has the small risk of false positive and false negative results your doctor may have you undergo additional blood tests that cross check the tTG-IgA test.

Instead of the tTG-IgA test, your doctor may choose to use the Endomysial Antibody (EMA) test which detects the same target antigen as the tTG-IgA test.

The disadvantage to using either of these blood tests is that a doctor visit is required, a blood sample must be drawn, and you must currently be eating gluten for the test to be valid.

Antibody blood tests cannot provide a conclusive diagnosis of Celiac Disease on their own. If you test positive on the tTG-IgA test or the EMA test your doctor will likely request endoscopy.

The advantage to beginning with these tests is that they are less invasive and less costly than endoscopy, requiring only a blood sample. If you test negative for tTG-IgA or EMA and negative on other blood tests that cross check these tests you most likely will not have to undergo endoscopy.

It is worth noting that patients who appear to be sensitive to gluten but who have not progressed to Celiac Disease (intestinal damage) may not test conclusively on one or more of these blood tests. In this case the patient may have to undergo additional testing as determined by their doctor.

Genetic Testing

Genetic tests are mildly invasive or non-invasive tests that are performed using an easily-obtained tissue sample whose DNA is scanned by a device called a genetic sequencer.

Genetic testing used to be expensive but rapidly advancing technology has driven the price down considerably, making it affordable for everyone.

While some genetic tests require blood to be drawn (necessitating a doctor visit), other genetic tests use a tissue sample that is taken in the privacy of the patient's home.

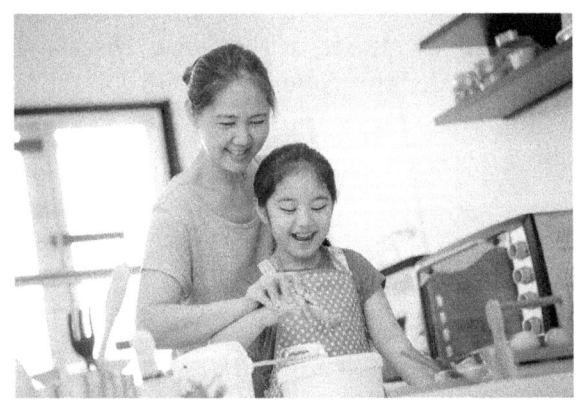

Genetic testing is often a shortcut for those whose relatives have been diagnosed with Celiac Disease

Some genetic tests use a large cotton swab to rub off cells from the interior of the patient's mouth (cheek swab test). The swab is then sent to the testing lab and results are given by mail or email. Other genetic tests use a saliva sample that the patient spits into a tube and sends to the testing lab.

With the advent of inexpensive genetic testing many patients have the option of having their DNA tested to determine if they carry one or more genes associated with Celiac Disease.

It is important to note that genetic testing cannot formally diagnose Celiac Disease. It can only predict whether you have the genetic predisposition to being unable to tolerate gluten. And just like those who carry genes that may predispose them to developing breast cancer but never develop breast cancer, those who carry genes that are associated with the inability to tolerate gluten may not express those genes (i.e. exhibit symptoms of gluten intolerance).

As such, genetic testing isn't for everyone but it is often a shortcut for those who have a close relative who has been diagnosed with Celiac Disease which is a hereditary disease. Those with a first-degree relative (parent, sibling, or child) who has been diagnosed with Celiac Disease have a 1 in 10 chance of developing Celiac Disease.

If the patient has a close family member who is a celiac, the patient displays symptoms of gluten intolerance that go away when the patient stops consuming gluten, and the patient tests positive for one or more genes associated with Celiac Disease then it is likely that the patient needs to adopt a gluten free diet for life.

Your doctor may still want to pursue antibody testing and endoscopy to further confirm gluten intolerance but many doctors are accepting results of genetic testing as sufficient evidence that the patient's symptoms are caused by gluten intolerance.

The advantage to using genetic tests is that they are inexpensive and only mildly invasive or non-invasive. In addition, the tests are accurate whether the patient is consuming gluten or has gone on a gluten-free diet. DNA sequencing does not measure antibodies that are produced in reaction to gluten so the patient may choose to go gluten-free prior to submitting their sample for genetic testing.

The disadvantage to using genetic tests is that they cannot formally diagnose Celiac Disease (which is diagnosed by endoscopy) and they can't predict whether patients who have no symptoms will express the genes for gluten intolerance at a later date.

Gluten Challenge Testing

A gluten challenge test is a method of testing for gluten intolerance that requires a patient to intentionally eat gluten to stimulate the patient's body to produce antibodies in sufficient quantity that the antibodies can be measured with antibody blood tests.

At first observation this method of testing seems illogical. If the patient already suspects that they cannot tolerate gluten and has seen a correlation between eating gluten-filled foods and pain and discomfort, then why would the patient intentionally put themselves through this discomfort to allow the doctor to measure the level of their antibodies?

It is a valid observation and many people forego this method of testing, choosing instead to undergo genetic testing which is at its worst case only mildly invasive and does not require the patient to be consuming gluten prior to testing. But genetic testing has its deficiencies. As mentioned previously, genetic testing cannot give a positive diagnosis of Celiac Disease and it can't predict whether a patient will express the genes that predispose them to Celiac Disease.

Patients are justified in their hesitation to undergo a gluten challenge test. When you consider that many doctors prescribe a measured amount of gluten that equals as many as 5 slices of wheat bread daily for 6 to 8 weeks, it is understandable why many patients hesitate when they are asked by their doctor to undergo a gluten challenge test.

At the end of the gluten challenge test your doctor will perform antibody blood testing. An endoscopy with biopsy (tissue sample) may be performed if the blood tests indicate antibodies were produced in sufficient number to indicate a positive test result.

The advantage of undergoing a gluten challenge test is that the doctor has a very controlled environment from which they can assess the patient's reaction to a specific level of gluten for a specific time period. This method of testing has little advantages for the patient, other than creating the environment from which their doctor can, with high confidence, conclusively diagnose Celiac Disease (if applicable to the patient).

The obvious disadvantage is that the patient may suffer considerably during the duration of the gluten challenge, which can be as long 8 weeks.

A secondary disadvantage is that a gluten challenge yields no conclusions on its own, it must be paired (at a minimum) with antibody blood tests. If the antibody blood tests are positive then the patient usually undergoes an endoscopy with biopsy to complete or rule out a diagnosis of Celiac Disease.

In the last few years, the medical community, realizing that the gluten challenge test is a slow and painful test for many patients, has strived to develop and accept a test that requires the patient to ingest gluten for a much shorter duration.

New tests in development require the patient to drink a measured amount of a gluten-containing drink. The patient's blood is drawn several hours later and is examined for presence of specific cytokines (proteins excreted by cells due to inflammation) that are associated with Celiac Disease.

While a shortened gluten challenge test can not lead to a diagnosis of Celiac Disease on its own, if approved by the medical community in the future, it can replace antibody blood tests which require the patient to be consuming gluten for a significant time period prior to the test.

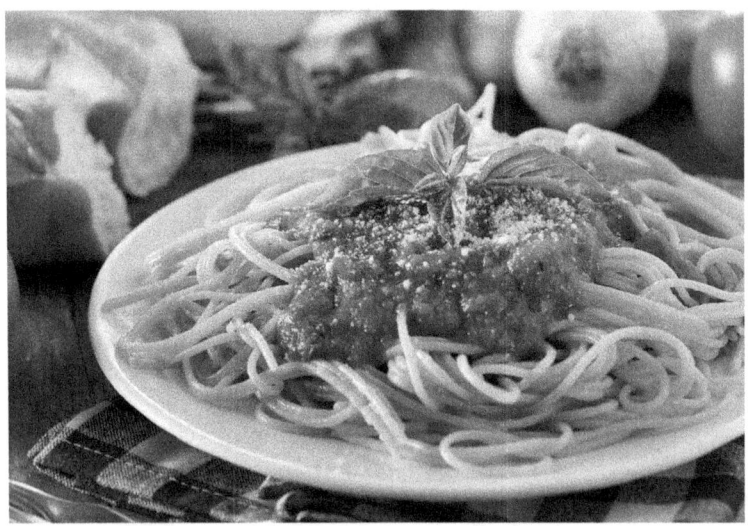

A gluten challenge test will require you to intentionally eat gluten for a specific time period

Methods of testing for gluten intolerance and Celiac Disease are evolving rapidly. Talk to your doctor about latest testing methods.

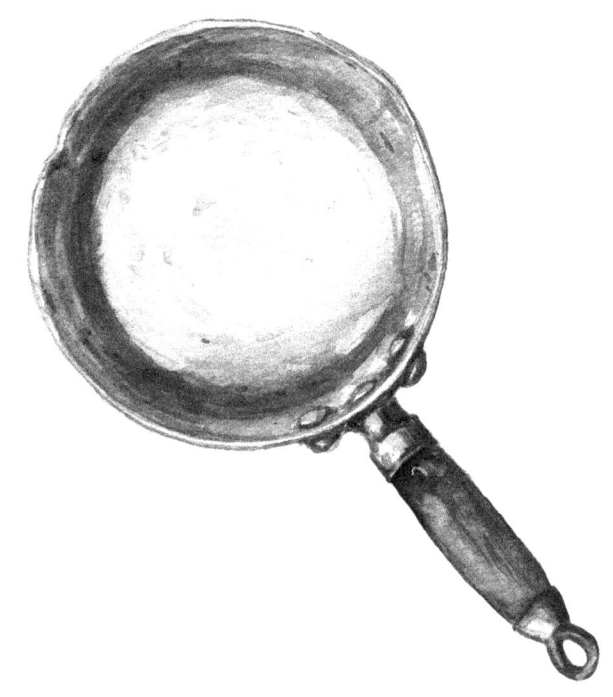

Cookware and Utensils

The recipes in this cookbook will require the use of some or all of the cookware and utensils listed on the following pages.

The two pieces of cookware that are necessary to make these recipes are a 12-inch (30.5 cm) skillet with lid and a 6-quart stockpot with lid.

Selecting a skillet

To determine skillet size look for a marking on the bottom of the skillet or measure the diameter of the skillet across the top of the skillet.

A smaller skillet such as a 10-inch skillet will not be big enough as these recipes are sized to almost completely fill the volume of a 12-inch skillet. If you have a slightly larger skillet (such as a 14-inch skillet) the recipe will likely succeed although cooking times may be affected.

You can use a skillet that is aluminum, cast iron, or coated with a non-stick finish which will make cleanup easier.

A useful feature is a see-through tempered glass lid which allows you to monitor the food without removing the lid.

Some lids have a vent hole for steam. If your skillet lid has a vent hole you may have to add a few more tablespoons of liquid to fully cook gluten-free pasta or rice used in the recipe.

Selecting a stockpot

To determine stockpot size look for a marking on the bottom of the stockpot that states the volume in quarts.

While a 6-quart stockpot is the preferred size for these recipes if you have a larger stockpot such as an 8-quart stockpot you may substitute your larger stockpot.

If your stockpot is coated with a non-stick finish that will make cleanup easier. A useful feature is a see-through tempered glass lid which allows you to monitor the food without removing the lid.

Other kitchen tools

The following kitchen tools and utensils may be necessary to prepare the recipes in this cookbook. It is not necessary to purchase professional-grade equipment but do consider buying the best quality knives your budget will allow as they are an investment that will pay off over decades of use.

Plastic cutting board

You will need a plastic cutting board. Do not use wood or bamboo cutting boards (see information on cross-contamination that follows). If you do not own a plastic cutting board then purchase one, preferably one that is dishwasher-safe. This will make cleanup and sterilization easier.

Many plastic cutting boards have features such as a non-skid backing to keep the cutting board from slipping while you chop foods. Others have a well around the perimeter of the board that acts as a moat to contain juices from meats and fruits.

These features are handy but not necessary. The only requirement is that the cutting board is not wood, bamboo, or some other porous and difficult to clean material.

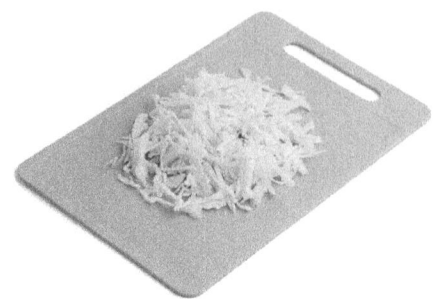

Plastic cutting board

Knives

A chef's knife is a medium-sized, general all-purpose knife that is used for slicing meats and chopping vegetables. A paring knife is a small knife that is used for peeling foods, trimming bits of fat from meat, or finely dicing vegetables such as onions.

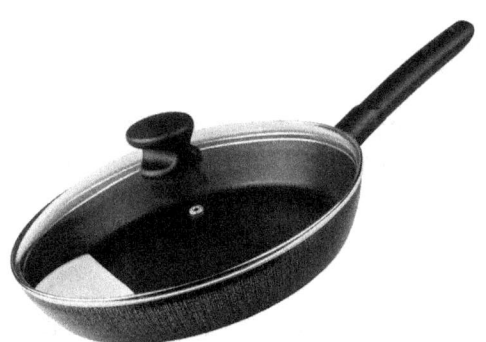
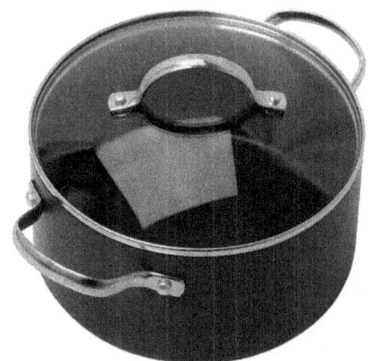

Left: Non-stick skillet with glass lid
Right: Non-stick stockpot with glass lid

If your budget can accommodate only one knife purchase then choose the chef's knife which is identified by its long, triangular blade.

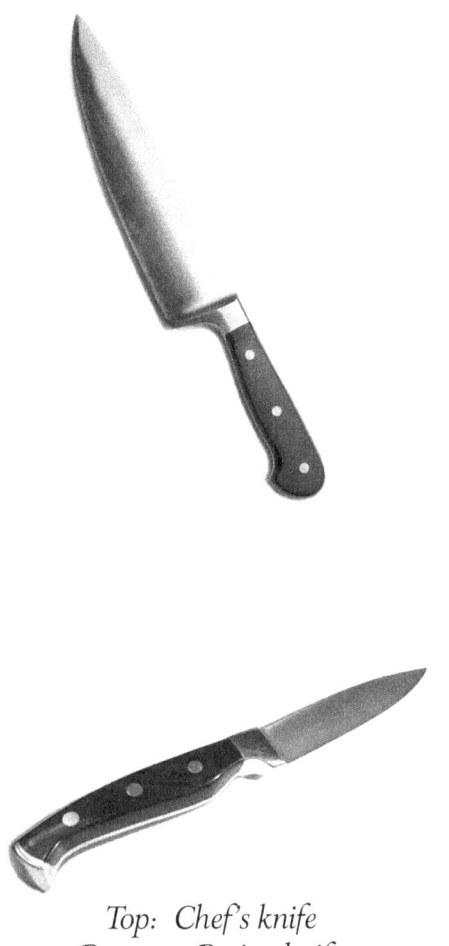

Top: Chef's knife
Bottom: Paring knife

For measuring and mixing foods

Many of the recipes in this cookbook give instructions to measure a portion of water and heat it in the microwave prior to its addition to the skillet or stockpot. This pre-heating is optional and is done to reduce cooking time.

If your liquid measuring cups are not microwave-safe (such as most plastic liquid measuring cups) then you may want to transfer the water to a microwave-safe bowl or you can simply add the unheated water directly into the skillet or stockpot.

Microwave-safe liquid measuring cups are made of heat-resistant glass and come in many sizes. The most common sizes are the 1-cup, 2-cup (pint), and 4-cup (quart) sizes.

If your budget allows the purchase of only one microwave-safe liquid measuring cup then the most useful size will be the 2-cup (pint) size.

For our purposes all the solid ingredients used in these recipes (such as rice and chopped vegetables) can be measured in clear liquid measuring cups which will provide reasonably accurate measures.

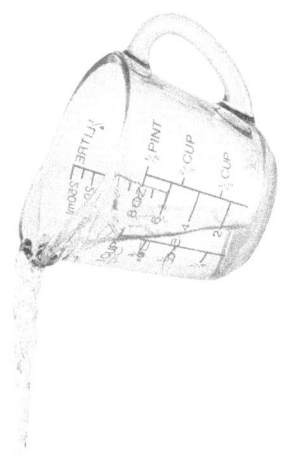

Microwave-safe
liquid measuring cup

You do not need to invest in a separate set of solid ingredient measuring cups if you do not have them. Solid ingredient measuring cups have a flat top edge that is useful for leveling foods, giving a more accurate measure.

Many of these recipes require pre-mixing of dry seasonings before addition to the skillet or stockpot. To pre-mix seasonings choose a small mixing bowl that holds a volume of one to two cups. Carefully measure the dry seasonings and add them directly into the small mixing bowl. Stir thoroughly to combine them before adding the mixed seasonings to the skillet or stockpot.

Cookware and Utensils

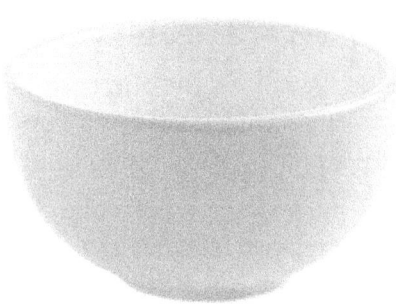

Small mixing bowl

You will need a set of metal or plastic measuring spoons to measure seasonings such as herbs and spices.

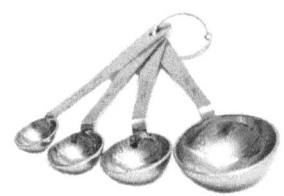

Set of measuring spoons

The recipes in this cookbook are given in the English measuring system (non-Metric). A standard set of measuring spoons will contain the following spoons:

Volume	Abbreviation	Metric Equivalent
1 tablespoon (3 teaspoons)	1 TBSP	15 ml
1 teaspoon	1 tsp	5 ml
1/2 teaspoon	1/2 tsp	2.5 ml
1/4 teaspoon	1/4 tsp	1.25 ml

For recipes that call for 1/8 teaspoon of seasoning use the 1/4 teaspoon measuring spoon and do your best to estimate one half of the volume of that measuring spoon.

Note that the American tablespoon is equal to 3 teaspoons while the Australian tablespoon is equal to 4 teaspoons. The recipes in this cookbook use the American tablespoon (3 teaspoons).

The seasonings in these recipes have been carefully adjusted for good overall flavor so it is important that you accurately measure each seasoning by leveling the top of the measuring spoon.

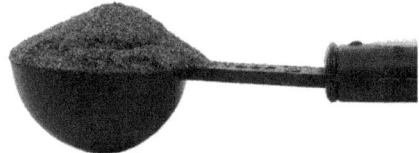

Level the top of the measuring spoon for an accurate measure

To measure dry seasonings use the measuring spoon to scoop the seasoning from its container. Hold the spoonful of seasoning over the container and take the flat edge of a butter knife and draw it across the top edge of the measuring spoon. This will level off the top of the mounded seasoning and allow the unused seasoning to drop back into the container.

For canned goods

Some of the recipes in this cookbook make use of canned vegetables or canned fish so you will need a can opener. A manual (non-electric) can opener will be adequate but if you like the convenience and don't mind spending the extra money you can purchase an electric can opener.

Whether you use a manual or electric can opener, remember to rinse and towel dry the cutting mechanism after each use to avoid cross-contamination (many canned products such as cream soups contain gluten).

NOTE: If your can opener is electric then you will need to remove the cutting mechanism from the body of the can opener before rinsing to avoid getting water into the can opener's electrical circuits. Dry the cutting mechanism thoroughly before reattaching it to the body of the can opener.

For rinsing and draining

Some recipes will require draining and rinsing of canned goods and other foods. A large-hole colander is best if you have one but you may substitute a fine mesh sieve.

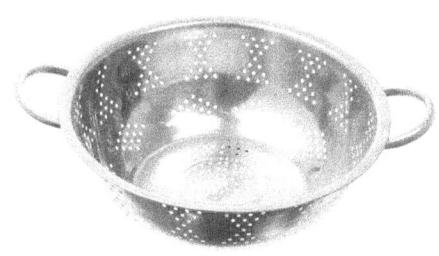

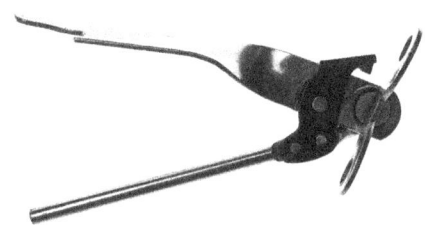

Manual can opener

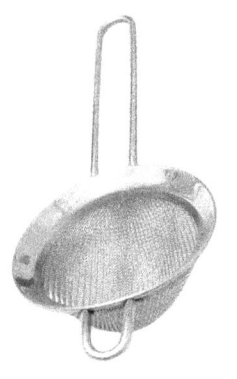

Top: colander
Bottom: mesh sieve

For shredding and grating

Many of the recipes in this cookbook use shredded or grated cheese. A shredder/grater will be necessary unless you plan to purchase pre-shredded and pre-grated cheeses.

The utensil's face that has the larger holes is useful for shredding medium density cheeses such as Cheddar and Mozzarella. The face that has the small holes can be used to grate hard cheeses such as Parmesan and Romano.

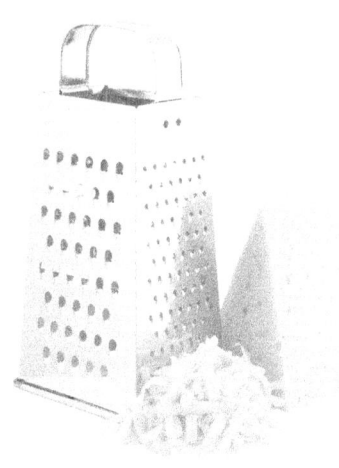

A shredder/grater is used to shred and grate cheese

Cookware and Utensils 47

For extracting juice

A citrus juicer is useful for extracting the juice from lemons, limes, and other citrus fruits. For best results position the juicer over a liquid measuring cup as shown. Slice the citrus fruit in half and place the halved fruit cut side down over the juicer. Press down on the halved fruit using a twisting motion to squeeze the juice from the pulp.

If you don't have a citrus juicer you can extract the juice by squeezing the halved fruit (cut side down) in the palm of your hand over a small bowl.

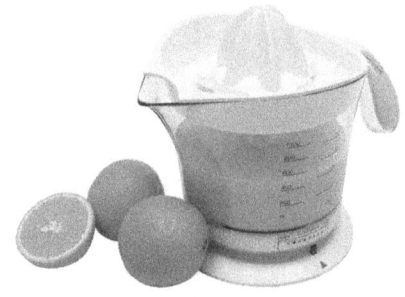

A citrus juicer extracts juice from citrus fruits

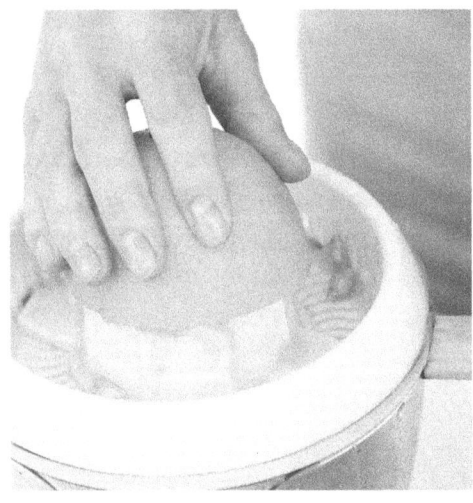

Use a twisting motion to squeeze juice from the pulp

Cross-contamination

Cross-contamination is the unintentional addition of gluten to normally gluten-free foods. It can occur at the manufacturer during processing of the food but it can also occur in restaurants and in your kitchen during food preparation.

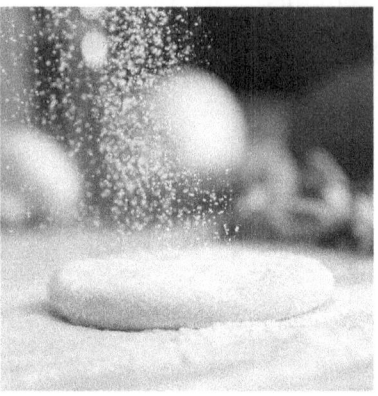

Cross-contamination can occur when wheat flour becomes airborne

Cross-contamination commonly occurs when wheat flour gets kicked up into the air during food preparation. This gluten-filled cloud of flour can settle on and contaminate gluten-free food so keep your food far away from stray flour.

Another cross-contamination risk is from bread crumbs. Non-gluten-free bread crumbs left on a cutting board or on a grill can get into your gluten-free food. To avoid stray bread crumbs, clean the grill or cutting board before making your meal.

Cross-contamination can also occur when using a cooking or serving utensil that was previously used to mix or serve a gluten-containing food. If the utensil isn't cleaned before preparing or serving your food then you may get a dose of gluten.

Wooden cookware and utensils

Wooden and bamboo cutting boards, bowls, and utensils can retain trace amounts of gluten-containing foods in the pores of the wood. If you are making a regular (gluten-containing) cake for a friend's birthday and you use a wooden spoon or wooden bowl then you risk the chance of residual gluten clinging to the pores of the spoon or bowl. The next time you use that bowl or spoon you may contaminate your own gluten-free birthday cake.

The remedy is to use only non-porous cookware and utensils made from plastic, glass, metal, or ceramic.

Invest in a plastic cutting board to chop foods. Plastic is non-porous and a trip through the dishwasher will restore the cutting board to an uncontaminated condition even if your friends decide to cut their baguette on it. The crumbs and flour will wash clean in the dishwasher and it will be good as new.

Mixing and serving utensils

Throw out all your wooden and bamboo mixing spoons, spatulas, and salad tongs. You can keep your 'single-use' wooden chop sticks and barbecue skewers as long as you don't contaminate them with gluten before use.

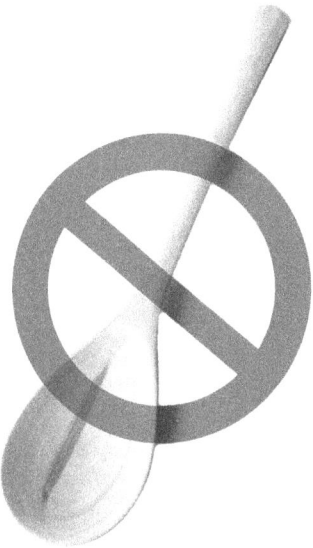

Throw away your wooden and bamboo utensils

Replace your multi-use wooden and bamboo utensils with heat-resistant plastic or metal utensils which will come clean in the dishwasher if they inadvertently become contaminated with gluten. You can use large-bowl spoons made from heat-resistant plastic such as the one shown below for stirring, mixing, and serving. An added bonus is that the plastic won't scratch non-stick cookware.

Throw away your wooden or bamboo cutting boards and use only plastic cutting boards

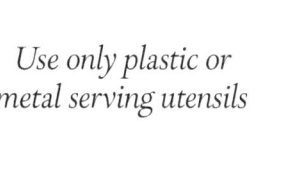

Use only plastic or metal serving utensils

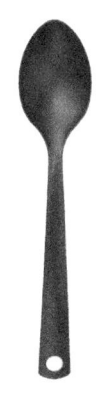

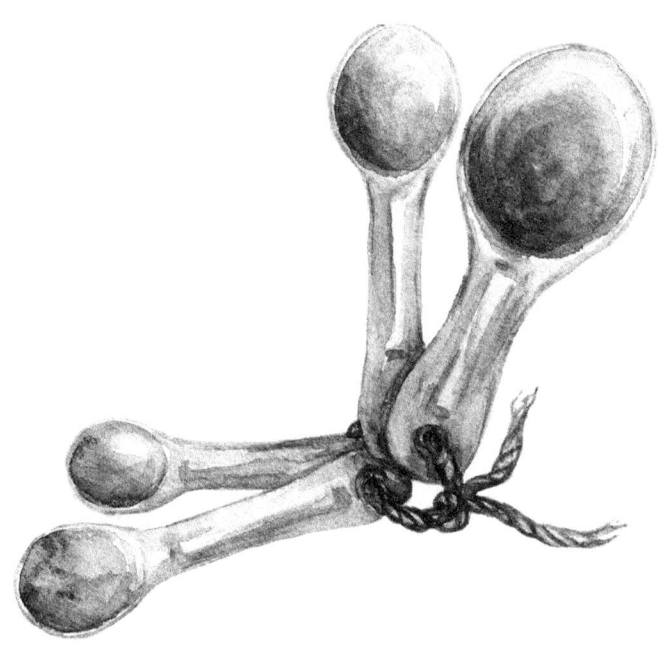

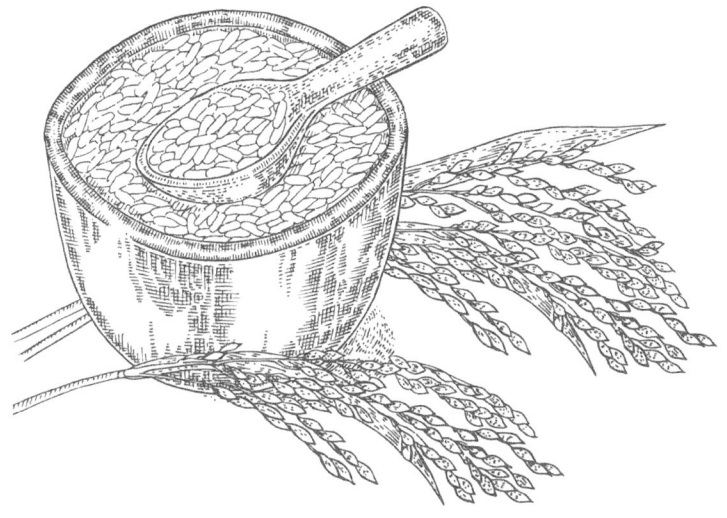

Converted Rice

Processed rice

Processed rice takes three forms: white rice, brown rice, and converted rice.

The most common type of processed rice is white rice. In white rice the husk, bran, and germ have been removed to expose the inner white grain. In the process of removing these outer components valuable vitamins and minerals are lost. White rice tends to become mushy if overcooked so cooking time must be carefully monitored.

Brown rice is a type of rice whose inedible husk has been removed but whose bran and germ have not been removed. Brown rice is more nutritious than white rice but takes longer to cook. Brown rice does not keep as long on your pantry shelf because the outer bran can become rancid.

Converted rice is also known as 'parboiled' rice because it is rice that has been partially boiled in its husk. After boiling the inedible husk is removed.

Parboiling draws nutrients into the core of the rice grain making parboiled rice nearly as nutritious as brown rice without the shorter shelf life. Converted (parboiled) rice also cooks quicker than brown rice but not as quickly as less-nutritious white rice.

An added benefit to using converted rice is that it holds its shape well when cooking, does not become mushy, and can withstand quite a bit of overcooking. This makes it an ideal substitute for white rice whose grains break down into a mush when overcooked.

Using converted rice

Many of the recipes in this cookbook call for the use of converted rice. You can find converted rice in the rice and grains section of your grocer.

Be sure to check that you are purchasing '100% converted rice' and not a flavored rice pilaf blend. Many large grocers and retailers sell their own inexpensive generic 'store label' brand of converted rice which can save you money.

If converted rice is not available you may substitute long-grain white rice but you may need to adjust the amount of liquid in the recipe to ensure complete cooking of the rice. You will also need to monitor the cooking time carefully so that the rice does not overcook and become mushy.

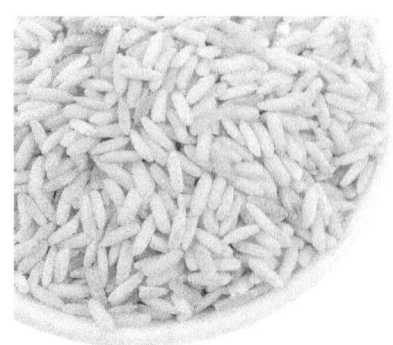

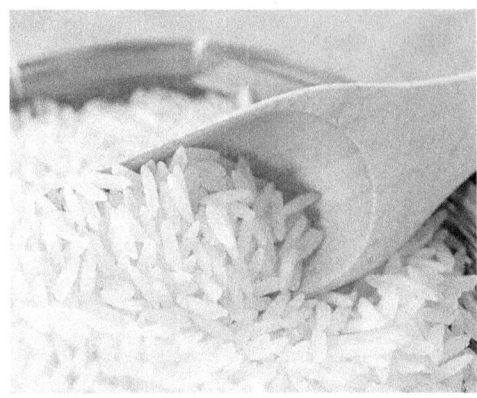

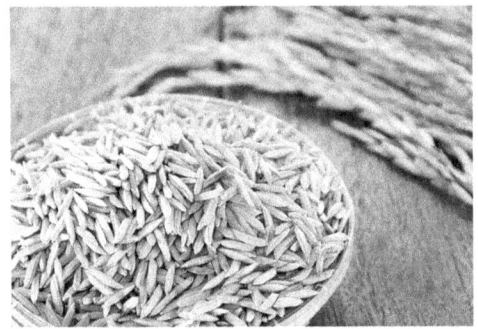

Unprocessed rice in husk

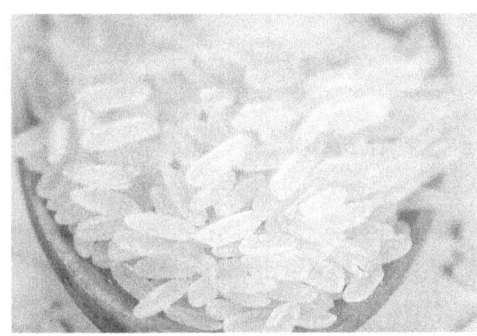

*Top to bottom:
Brown rice, white rice, converted rice*

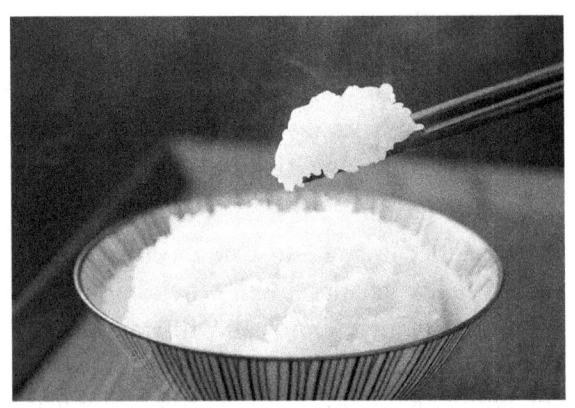

White rice can become mushy if overcooked

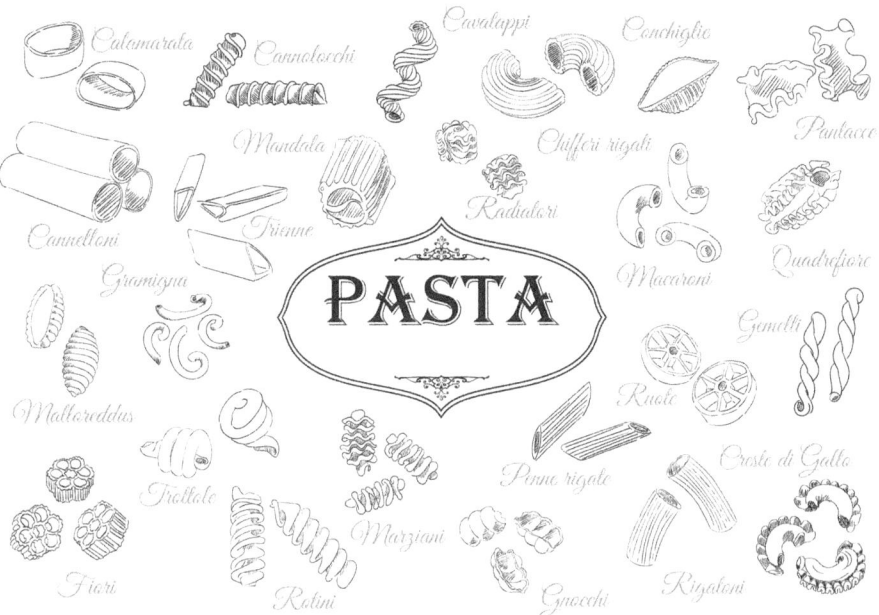

Measuring Pasta

Many of the recipes in this cookbook use gluten-free pasta as an ingredient. Gluten-free pasta can be made from rice, corn, quinoa, millet, amaranth, or other gluten-free grains.

Unless specifically stated otherwise in the ingredients list the recipes in this cookbook were formulated and tested using 100% rice pasta which was chosen for its ability to withstand over-cooking without becoming mushy as compared to pasta made from corn or other gluten-free grains.

If you use gluten-free pastas made from other grains (including rice blends) you may have varying results which can include shorter cooking times or the need for more or less liquid in the recipe.

Measuring gluten-free pasta

Pasta comes in many shapes and sizes. The size and shape of different types of pasta can vary considerably.

Because the size and shape of different types of pasta varies so much it is preferable to measure the pasta by weighing it rather than measuring by volume in a measuring cup. An ounce of spaghetti will absorb approximately the same amount of liquid as an ounce of penne pasta. It is easier to formulate a recipe that is universal for all types of pasta if the pasta is measured by weight.

In the past, those on a gluten-free diet were limited in the types of gluten-free pastas that were available. As little as ten years ago it was difficult to find anything but gluten-free spaghetti and elbow noodles.

Now it is easy to find gluten-free penne, lasagna noodles, rotini, egg noodles, linguini, fusilli, pasta shells, and even gluten-free ravioli in your grocer's refrigerated deli section.

The most readily available pasta shapes that are suitable for these recipes are elbow noodles, penne pasta, and rotini (corkscrew pasta). Most gluten-free pasta manufacturers offer one or more of these pasta shapes.

Measuring pasta by weight

Measuring pasta by weight is the most accurate way to determine the correct amount of pasta for these recipes.

Most of the recipes in this cookbook call for 8 ounces (227 grams) of pasta. In the United States most gluten-free pasta is sold in packages of 12 ounces or 16 ounces (1 pound). This means that you may use only a portion of the package for the recipe. Unused pasta can be stored in a plastic bag or airtight container for several months in your pantry.

To measure pasta by weight you will need a kitchen scale. If you don't have a kitchen scale you will need to estimate the weight of the pasta by its volume (see *Measuring by Volume*).

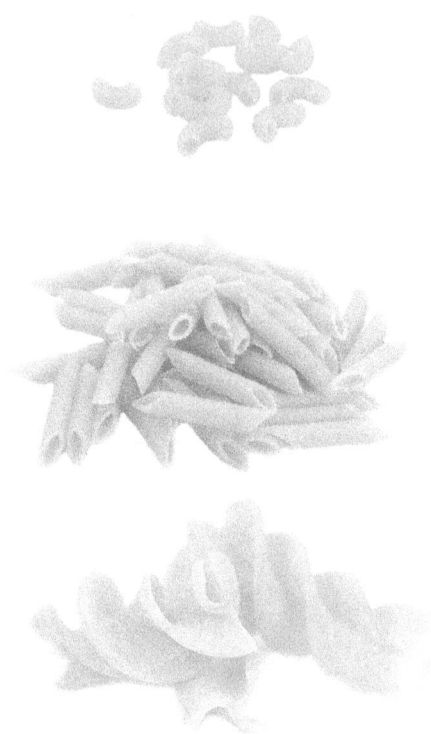

Top to bottom: elbow noodles, penne, rotini (corkscrew pasta)

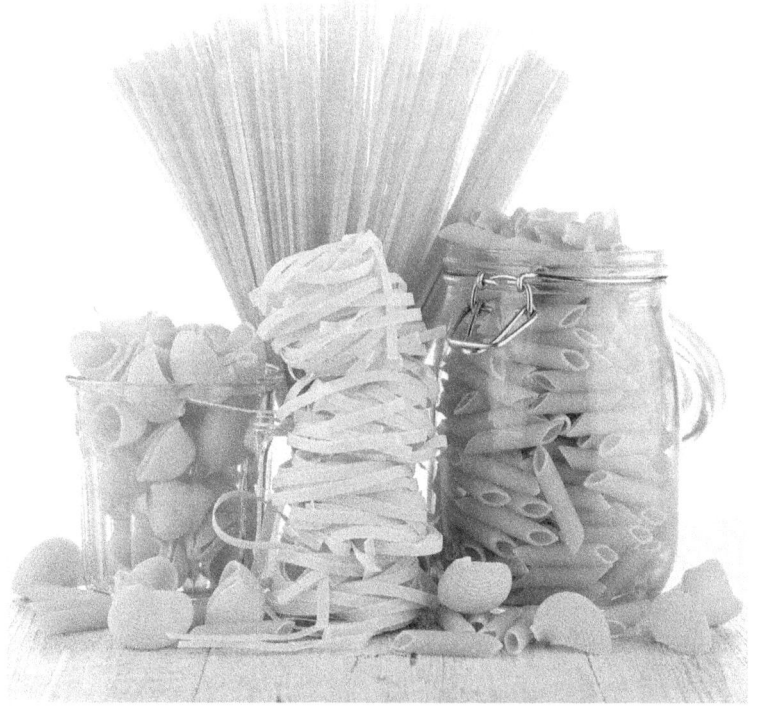

Gluten-free pasta comes in many shapes and sizes

Weighing the pasta

The first step in measuring the pasta is to tare (or 'zero') the scale with the empty measuring container on the scale.

Kitchen scales come in two varieties, digital and analog. You can tare a kitchen scale by the following methods:

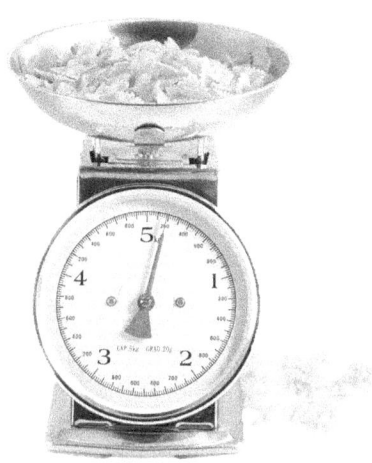

A kitchen scale is used to weigh pasta

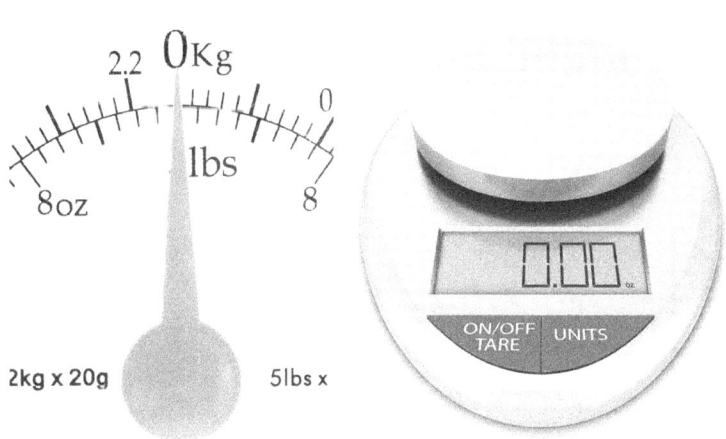

Tare (zero) the scale with the empty measuring container on the scale

For digital scales there will be a button labeled TARE that may or may not be combined with the ON/OFF button. Turn the scale on. Put the empty measuring container on the scale then press the TARE button until the scale reads zero.

For analog scales there will usually be a thumb dial or turn screw located on the body of the scale, often on the back side or near the bottom front face of the scale.

Put the empty measuring container on the scale then turn the thumb dial or turn screw until the scale reads zero. After you tare the scale you can transfer the pasta into the measuring container. Transfer the pasta slowly so you do not spill and so you don't overshoot the target weight.

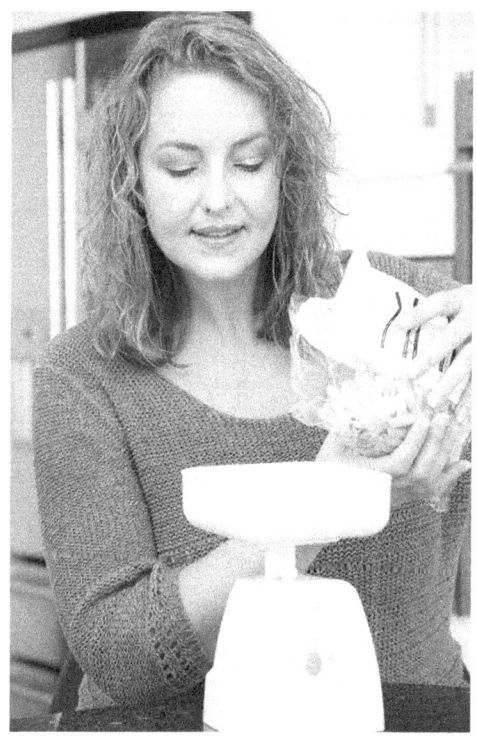

Carefully transfer the pasta to the measuring container

If you overshoot the target weight remove some of the pasta and note the new reading, repeating this process until you are at the target weight.

Measuring Pasta 55

Measuring by volume

If you do not have a kitchen scale you can estimate how much pasta you need by measuring the volume of the entire package then calculating the volume you need for the recipe as a fraction of the total package volume.

As a shortcut, use the following tables to estimate the volume (in cups) of 8 oz of pasta.

Store unused pasta in a plastic bag or airtight container in your pantry. Unused pasta will remain fresh for several months.

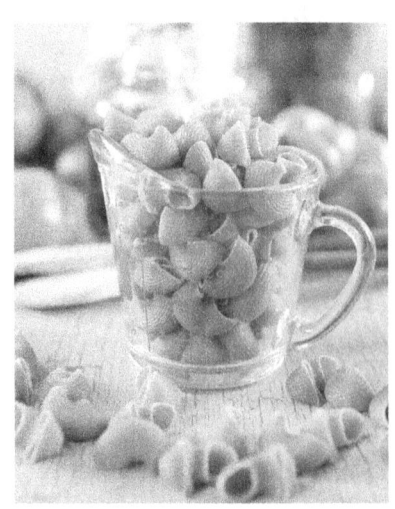

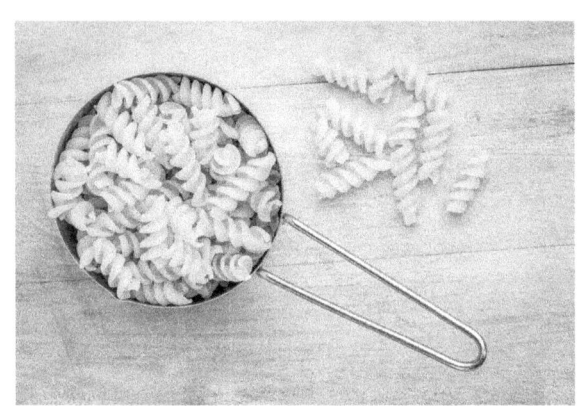

Clear and opaque measuring containers may be used to measure pasta by volume

For *12-oz packages* of pasta

Total Package Volume (12 oz)	Volume needed for recipe (8 oz)
6 cups	4 cups
5 1/2 cups	3 2/3 cups
5 cups	3 1/3 cups
4 1/2 cups	3 cups
4 cups	2 2/3 cups
3 1/2 cups	2 1/3 cups
3 cups	2 cups
2 1/2 cups	1 2/3 cups
2 cups	1 1/3 cups

For *16-oz packages* of pasta

Total Package Volume (16 oz)	Volume needed for recipe (8 oz)
6 cups	3 cups
5 1/2 cups	2 3/4 cups
5 cups	2 1/2 cups
4 1/2 cups	2 1/4 cups
4 cups	2 cups
3 1/2 cups	1 3/4 cups
3 cups	1 1/2 cups
2 1/2 cups	1 1/4 cups
2 cups	1 cup

Tips

Some of the ingredients used in the recipes in this cookbook are processed foods whose ingredients list must be carefully examined to ensure that the product contains no gluten. Below are some tips for selecting processed foods that are safe for consumption.

Shredded or grated cheese

Manufacturers who make shredded or grated cheeses often coat the cheese with a powder to keep the cheese from clumping. In the past some manufacturers have used wheat flour as an anti-clumping agent.

Fortunately, most shredded or grated cheeses now contain gluten-free anti-caking agents such as potato starch, corn starch, or powdered cellulose (commonly made from wood pulp).

If the product is made in the United States and the allergen information does not list WHEAT then the starch is usually safe.

If you are extremely sensitive to cross-contamination that can be introduced during the manufacturing process then buy bulk cheese and shred it yourself.

Garlic

Garlic is available as a seasoning in many forms: fresh bulbs and cloves, garlic juice, dried garlic flakes (minced garlic), granulated garlic, garlic powder, and garlic flavored salt (garlic salt).

Many of the recipes in this cookbook use granulated garlic as a seasoning instead of fresh garlic which has a shorter shelf life. Fresh garlic must also be peeled and chopped which increases preparation time.

Unless fresh garlic is specified always use granulated garlic in these recipes. Do not substitute garlic salt as the dish will taste too salty.

You can identify granulated garlic by its sand-like, gritty texture. Garlic powder is similar but has a flour-like consistency and will be too concentrated, resulting in an overly-intense garlic flavor.

Garlic powder is also likely to contain additives (some of which may not be gluten-free) that are used to improve flow and prevent clumping.

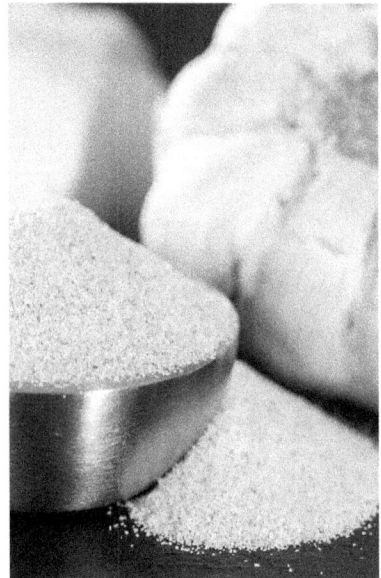

Granulated garlic has a gritty sand-like texture

Store granulated garlic in your pantry in a tightly sealed glass or plastic jar away from light, heat, and humidity. With proper storage granulated garlic will remain fresh in your pantry for a year or more.

Broth

Before the benefits of a gluten-free diet were widely known it was difficult to find a packaged broth that did not contain gluten or MSG (mono sodium glutamate), an ingredient that many people who must follow a gluten-free diet are also sensitive to.

Now many grocers offer broths made without gluten-containing ingredients that are packaged in handy, quart-sized boxes that do not need to be refrigerated until opened.

If possible, select a broth that does not contain MSG. Review the ingredients list carefully for any ingredients that could contain gluten.

Many manufacturers are now making their broths gluten-free. If you are sensitive to cross-contamination that can occur during the manufacturing process then select a broth that is labeled gluten-free.

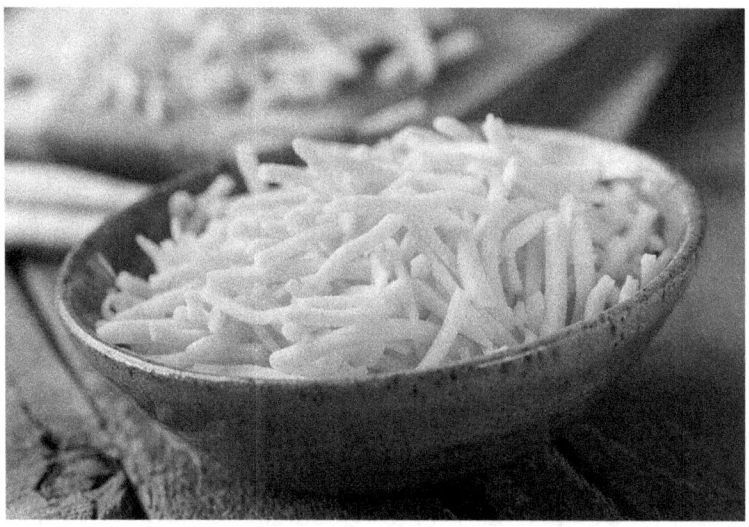

Pre-packaged shredded or grated cheeses can contain gluten

Unused broth can be refrigerated for up to week or frozen for up to a month. Before freezing, transfer the unused broth to a plastic or glass container. The boxed broths often use a package that is lined with metal foil which is not suitable for thawing in the microwave.

Non-fat dry milk

Non-fat dry milk is a powdered form of milk whose fat has been removed prior to dehydrating. In addition to being convenient, low-cost, and storable on your pantry shelf it is a healthy substitute for regular milk. Non-fat dry milk can be used in place of regular milk in all the recipes in this cookbook.

In the United States many brands of non-fat dry milk are sold in convenient pouches designed to reconstitute into one quart of milk.

If you have a 1-quart (4-cup) liquid measuring pitcher simply empty the pouch of powdered milk into the pitcher and add cold water until the liquid reaches the 1-quart line. Stir until all powder has been reconstituted. Store unused reconstituted milk in the refrigerator for up to three days.

Non-fat dry milk is healthy, inexpensive, and convenient

Wheat-free Tamari Sauce (soy sauce substitute)

Most brands of soy sauce contain wheat as an ingredient. Wheat-free Tamari Sauce is a gluten-free alternative to soy sauce that has a richer, earthier flavor.

Be sure to select a brand of Tamari Sauce that is specifically labeled 'wheat-free' or 'gluten-free'. Wheat-free tamari sauce can be found at well-stocked grocers and Asian markets.

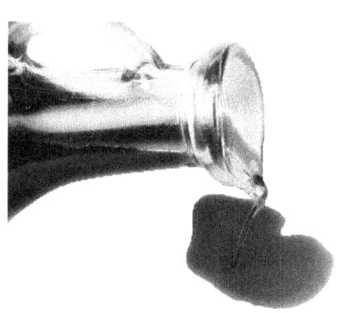

Wheat-free Tamari Sauce is a substitute for soy sauce

Canned fish

In the past, many canned tunas and other types of water-packed canned fish were flavored with broths that contained wheat. It is becoming more common for canned tuna to be flavored with vegetable broths, usually soy flavoring. Some manufacturers have eliminated the flavorings and are packing their canned fish in a salt and water brine.

Read the ingredients list carefully when selecting water-packed canned fish. When possible, select canned fish that has been labeled gluten-free. Avoid soy-based broths if you are allergic to soy.

If you are unable to find water-packed gluten-free tuna you can substitute oil-packed tuna. Drain the oil-packed tuna in a metal sieve. Rinse the fish gently with a hot water spray to rinse away the oil. Allow the excess water to drain before using.

Seasoning Blends

Some of the recipes in this cookbook use Chili Powder, Taco Seasoning, and other seasoning blends that may have a starch added to prevent clumping.

In the United States if the ingredients list specifies corn starch, potato starch, or modified food starch and the allergen information does not list WHEAT then the seasoning is usually safe for consumption.

If you are extremely sensitive to cross-contamination with gluten then select a seasoning blend that is labeled 'gluten-free'.

Sour cream and yogurt

Some of the recipes in this cookbook call for the use of sour cream or unflavored (plain) yogurt. Many manufacturers of sour cream use modified food starch to thicken their product.

If the sour cream is manufactured in the United States then the food source for the starch will be corn so the product will not intentionally contain gluten. If you are extremely sensitive to gluten select a sour cream without added starch or one labeled 'gluten-free'.

Some yogurts use a starch as a thickening agent. This starch may contain gluten. Many manufacturers have been labeling their gluten-free yogurts making it relatively easy to select a yogurt that is safe for consumption. If you are not able to find a yogurt that is labeled gluten-free then select one without added starch.

Ground turkey

Some of the recipes in this cookbook allow the use of ground turkey as a substitute for ground beef. It is common for a seasoning to be added to flavor packaged ground turkey.

When substituting packaged ground turkey check the ingredients list carefully for seasonings that may contain gluten. If possible, select a packaged ground turkey that is labeled 'gluten-free' or buy unseasoned ground turkey directly from your butcher.

Ham and sausage

In the past, gluten-containing starches and flavorings were often added as a filler to processed hams and sausages to inexpensively increase the volume of the product.

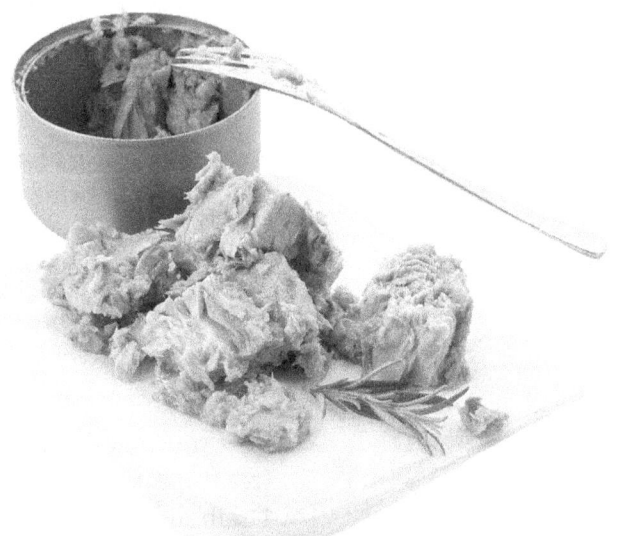

Some types of canned fish can contain gluten

Thankfully, in the United States the use of wheat starch and other gluten-containing grains has declined. The exception is ethnic specialty sausages which can contain barley to stay true to their traditional recipe.

If you are unable to find ham or sausage products that are labeled 'gluten-free' then check the ingredients list carefully for gluten. If the product is manufactured in the United States, the ingredients list does not list WHEAT, BARLEY, or RYE as an ingredient, and the allergen information does not list WHEAT then the processed meat is usually safe to eat.

MSG (mono sodium glutamate) is an ingredient that many people who must follow a gluten-free diet are also sensitive to. Some processed meats contain MSG. If you are sensitive to MSG then select a processed meat product that does not contain this additive.

Worcestershire Sauce

Many brands of Worcestershire Sauce contain wheat. When purchasing Worcestershire Sauce read the ingredients list carefully to ensure that wheat is not listed as an ingredient.

Clam juice

Clam juice is made by steaming clams and extracting their juice. It usually does not contain gluten but it may contain MSG (mono sodium glutamate), an ingredient that many people who must follow a gluten-free diet are also sensitive to. If you are sensitive to MSG then select a brand of clam juice that does not contain this additive.

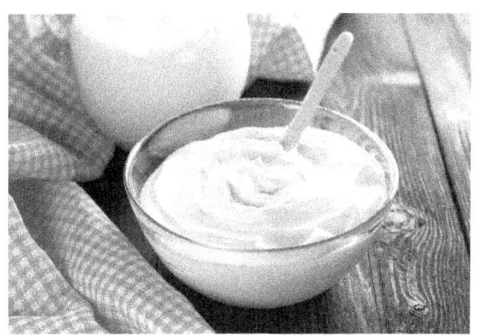

Sour cream and yogurt may contain gluten

Metric Conversion

All of the recipes in this cookbook are given in English (Imperial) measurements. If your measuring equipment is sized for the metric system then use the following tables to convert from the English system (pounds, ounces, cups) to the metric system (liters, milliliters, grams).

Measurement

CUP	ONCES	MILLILITERS	TABLESPOONS
8 cup	64 oz	1895 ml	128
6 cup	48 oz	1420 ml	96
5 cup	40 oz	1180 ml	80
4 cup	32 oz	960 ml	64
2 cup	16 oz	480 ml	32
1 cup	8 oz	240 ml	16
3/4 cup	6 oz	177 ml	12
2/3 cup	5 oz	158 ml	11
1/2 cup	4 oz	118 ml	8
3/8 cup	3 oz	90 ml	6
1/3 cup	2.5 oz	79 ml	5.5
1/4 cup	2 oz	59 ml	4
1/8 cup	1 oz	30 ml	3
1/16 cup	1/2 oz	15 ml	1

Temperature

FAHRENHEIT	CELSIUS
100 °F	37 °C
150 °F	65 °C
200 °F	93 °C
250 °F	121 °C
300 °F	150 °C
325 °F	160 °C
350 °F	180 °C
375 °F	190 °C
400 °F	200 °C
425 °F	220 °C
450 °F	230 °C
500 °F	260 °C
525 °F	274 °C
550 °F	288 °C

Weight

IMPERIAL	METRIC
1/2 oz	15 g
1 oz	29 g
2 oz	57 g
3 oz	85 g
4 oz	113 g
5 oz	141 g
6 oz	170 g
8 oz	227 g
10 oz	283 g
12 oz	340 g
13 oz	369 g
14 oz	397 g
15 oz	425 g
1 lb	453 g

Metric conversions for temperature and weight

Beef and Lamb

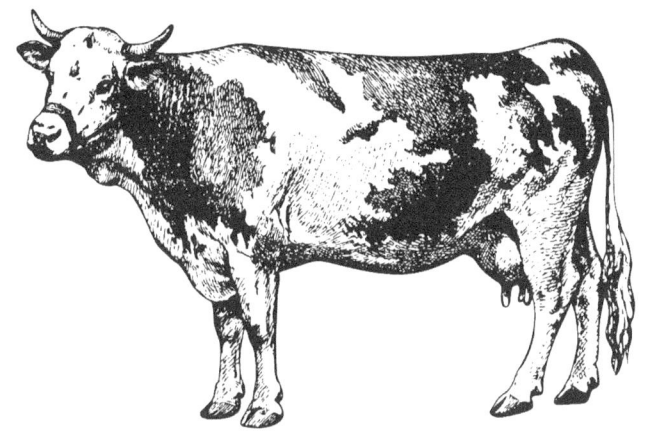

Meals in a Skillet

- 64 Taco in a Skillet
- 65 Beefy Italian Skillet
- 66 Chili Macaroni Skillet
- 67 Asian Beef and Broccoli Skillet
- 68 Hungarian Goulash Skillet
- 69 Original Hamburger Macaroni Skillet
- 70 Greek Skillet with Olives and Feta
- 71 Salisbury Beef and Mushroom Skillet
- 72 Mexican Beef and Rice Skillet
- 73 Cheeseburger Macaroni Skillet
- 74 Beef Stew in a Skillet
- 75 Stroganoff Mushroom Skillet
- 76 Skillet Shepherd's Pie
- 78 Skillet Tamale Pie

Soups and Stews

- 80 Savory Beef Stew with Winter Vegetables
- 81 Classic Beef Chili
- 82 Gluten-Free Cornbread Muffins
- 84 Easy Vegetable Beef Soup
- 85 Saucy Cabbage and Hamburger Soup
- 86 October Cider Stew
- 87 Herbed French (Italian) Onion Soup
- 88 Mediterranean Lamb Stew
- 89 Stuffed Pepper Soup
- 90 Easy Vietnamese Pho
- 92 Hot and Smoky Beer and Bacon Chili
- 93 Herbed Provencal Beef Stew

Taco in a Skillet

This zesty skillet combines all the flavors of a taco dinner in one dish – beef, corn, tomatoes, Cheddar cheese, onions, and peppers. Choose the heat (hot, medium, mild) of the prepared salsa used in the recipe to suit your taste.

Ingredients

1 lb ground beef
1 cup onion, chopped
  (about 1/2 of a large onion)
2 cups water, heated
2 TBSP taco seasoning *
1 16-oz jar tomato salsa (red salsa)
8 oz gluten-free pasta **
1 cup shredded Cheddar cheese *
  (about 4 oz by weight)
1 cup frozen corn kernels

* See **Tips** section
** See **Measuring Pasta** section

Cookware and Utensils

12-inch skillet with lid
Microwave-safe liquid measuring cup
  (2-cup size or larger)
Shredder/grater
  (if not using pre-shredded cheese)

Instructions

1. Add the ground beef to the skillet, breaking it into small chunks, about 3/4-inch in size. Cover the skillet with the lid. Brown the ground beef on medium heat.

2. While the ground beef is browning chop the onion. Add the chopped onion to the ground beef. Stir to combine.

3. Microwave 2 cups of water on high power for 2 minutes.

4. Check the ground beef for doneness. The ground beef is fully cooked when there is no pink color. Drain the fat if desired. This step is not necessary if a low-fat ground beef is used.

5. Sprinkle the taco seasoning over the cooked ground beef. Stir to coat the ground beef with the taco seasoning.

6. Add the prepared salsa to the ground beef mixture. Stir to combine.

7. Add the hot water to the ground beef and salsa mixture. Stir to combine.

8. Add the gluten-free pasta to the ground beef and salsa mixture. Stir to combine. Cover the skillet with the lid. Increase the heat to medium high until the mixture boils then reduce the heat to a gentle simmer.

9. Most gluten-free pastas cook in 7 to 12 minutes. Stir the mixture frequently, checking every 3 to 4 minutes until the pasta is cooked to your taste.

10. While the pasta is cooking shred the Cheddar cheese (if not using pre-shredded cheese).

11. When the pasta is cooked to the desired doneness stir in the frozen corn kernels. Cover the skillet with the lid and heat for a few minutes to thaw the frozen corn kernels.

12. Add the shredded cheese to the skillet. Stir to combine. Cover the skillet with the lid. Turn off the heat and allow the cheese to fully melt. Stir again to combine the cheese. Serve immediately.

Beefy Italian Skillet

This delicious skillet is loaded with beef, tomatoes, Italian herbs, and Parmesan cheese. It is an easy one-pot alternative to an ordinary spaghetti with meat sauce dinner.

Ingredients

1 lb ground beef
1 cup onion, chopped
  (about 1/2 of a large onion)
1 tsp salt
1 tsp basil, dried
1 1/2 tsp oregano, dried
2 tsp granulated garlic *
1/4 tsp black pepper
1/4 tsp hot red pepper flakes
1 cup water, heated
1 28-oz can tomatoes, diced or crushed
  (do not drain)
8 oz gluten-free pasta **
3/4 cup grated Parmesan cheese *

* See *Tips* section
** See *Measuring Pasta* section

Cookware and Utensils

12-inch skillet with lid
Small bowl
Microwave-safe liquid measuring cup
  (1-cup size or larger)
Shredder/grater
  (if not using pre-grated cheese)

Instructions

1. Add the ground beef to the skillet, breaking it into small chunks, about 3/4-inch in size. Cover the skillet with the lid. Brown the ground beef on medium heat.

2. While the ground beef is browning chop the onion. Add the chopped onion to the ground beef. Stir to combine.

3. Measure the salt, basil, oregano, garlic, black pepper, and red pepper flakes into a small bowl. Stir to combine.

4. Microwave 1 cup of water on high power for one minute.

5. Check the ground beef for doneness. The ground beef is fully cooked when there is no pink color. Drain the fat if desired (this step is not necessary if a low-fat ground beef is used).

6. Sprinkle the seasonings over the cooked ground beef. Stir to coat the ground beef with the seasonings.

7. Add the tomatoes (do not drain) and the hot water to the ground beef mixture. Stir to combine.

8. Add the gluten-free pasta to the beef and tomato mixture. Stir to combine. Cover the skillet with the lid. Increase the heat to medium high until the mixture boils then reduce the heat to a gentle simmer.

9. Most gluten-free pastas cook in 7 to 12 minutes. Stir the mixture frequently, checking every 3 to 4 minutes until the pasta is cooked to your taste.

10. While the pasta is cooking grate the Parmesan cheese (if not using pre-grated cheese).

11. When the pasta is cooked to the desired doneness sprinkle the grated cheese over the skillet. Serve immediately.

Chili Macaroni Skillet

A hot and spicy bowl of chili is a satisfying meal unto itself. This recipe pairs savory tomatoes and tangy Cheddar cheese with macaroni and beans for a quick and easy chili dinner.

Ingredients

1 lb ground beef
1 cup onion, chopped
  (about 1/2 of a large onion)
1/2 green bell pepper,
  seeded and diced into 1/2" pieces
1 TBSP chili powder *
1 tsp sugar
1 tsp salt
1 tsp granulated garlic *
1/2 tsp oregano, dried
2 cups water, heated
1 15-oz can tomatoes, diced or crushed
  (do not drain)
1/2 cup milk *
8 oz gluten-free pasta **
1 cup shredded Cheddar cheese *
  (about 4 oz by weight)
1 15-oz can black beans or red
  kidney beans, rinsed and drained

* See **Tips** section
** See **Measuring Pasta** section

Cookware and Utensils

12-inch skillet with lid
Small bowl
Microwave safe liquid measuring cup
  (2-cup size or larger)
Shredder/grater
  (if not using pre-shredded cheese)
Colander

Instructions

1. Add the ground beef to the skillet, breaking it into small chunks, about 3/4-inch in size. Cover the skillet with the lid. Brown the ground beef on medium heat.

2. While the ground beef is browning chop the onion and the bell pepper. Add the onion and bell pepper to the ground beef. Stir to combine.

3. Measure the chili powder, sugar, salt, garlic, and oregano into a small bowl. Stir to combine.

4. Microwave 2 cups of water on high power for 2 minutes.

5. Check the ground beef for doneness. The ground beef is fully cooked when there is no pink color. Drain the fat if desired (this step is not necessary if a low-fat ground beef is used). Sprinkle the seasonings over the cooked ground beef. Stir to coat the ground beef with the seasonings.

6. Add the tomatoes to the skillet (do not drain). Stir to combine.

7. Add the hot water and the milk to the skillet. Stir to combine.

8. Add the gluten-free pasta to the skillet. Stir to combine. Cover the skillet with the lid. Increase the heat to medium high until the mixture boils then reduce the heat to a gentle simmer. Stir occasionally. Most gluten-free pastas cook in 7 to 12 minutes. Stir the mixture frequently, checking every 3 to 4 minutes until the pasta is cooked to your taste.

9. While the pasta is cooking shred the Cheddar cheese (if not using pre-shredded cheese).

10. Rinse the beans in the colander and allow them to drain completely.

11. When the pasta is cooked to the desired doneness gently stir in the beans. Cover the skillet with the lid and heat for a few minutes to warm the beans.

12. Add the shredded cheese to the skillet. Stir to combine. Cover the skillet with the lid. Turn off the heat and allow the cheese to fully melt. Stir again to combine the cheese. Serve immediately.

Asian Beef and Broccoli Skillet

Many Asian dishes are naturally gluten-free and need no modification for those on a gluten-free diet. Dishes that use soy sauce are the exception as most soy sauces contain wheat. This recipe substitutes wheat-free Tamari sauce which is an earthier, richer-flavored type of soy sauce.

Ingredients

12 oz frozen broccoli florets
1 lb boneless sirloin steak,
  trimmed of fat,
  sliced thinly into 3/8" thick slices,
  slices cut into 2" lengths
3 TBSP vegetable oil
3 cups water, heated
1 tsp sugar
1/2 tsp ground ginger
1/2 tsp granulated garlic *
1 1/2 cups converted (parboiled) rice **
1/4 cup wheat-free Tamari Sauce *

* See *Tips* section
** See *Converted Rice* section

Cookware and Utensils

12-inch skillet with lid
Microwave-safe liquid measuring cup
  (3-cup size or larger)

Instructions

1. Remove the frozen broccoli florets from the freezer. Thaw them on the countertop while preparing the steak and rice mixture.

2. Trim the fat from the steak. Slice the steak thinly into 3/8-inch thick strips. Cut the strips into 2-inch lengths.

3. Add the steak and the vegetable oil to the skillet. Stir to combine. Stir fry the steak on medium high heat until it begins to lose its pink color. Stir frequently to prevent burning.

4. While the steak is cooking microwave 3 cups of water on high power for 3 minutes.

5. After the steak has lost its pink color reduce the heat to medium. Add the sugar, ginger, and garlic to the skillet. Stir to coat the steak with the seasonings.

6. Add the converted (parboiled) rice to the steak mixture. Stir to coat the rice with the seasonings.

7. Add the hot water and the Tamari Sauce to the steak and rice mixture. Stir to combine. Cover the skillet with the lid. Increase the heat to medium high until the mixture boils then reduce the heat to a gentle simmer. Stir occasionally.

8. When the rice is soft and the water is fully absorbed add the thawed broccoli florets to the skillet. Stir to combine. Cover the skillet with the lid and heat for a few minutes until the broccoli is tender crisp. Serve immediately.

Hungarian Goulash Skillet

Many Hungarian dishes feature paprika which is the main seasoning in this skillet. Choose a good quality Hungarian sweet paprika for the best flavor. It costs a little more than the bland supermarket paprika but the difference in taste is worth it.

Ingredients

1 lb ground beef or ground turkey *
1 cup onion, chopped
  (about 1/2 of a large onion)
1 green bell pepper,
  seeded and diced into 1/2" pieces
1 tsp sugar
1 tsp salt
1/2 tsp black pepper
1 1/2 tsp granulated garlic *
1/4 tsp caraway seed
1 TBSP Hungarian sweet paprika
1 8-oz can tomato sauce
2 cups gluten-free beef broth *
1 bay leaf
8 oz gluten-free pasta **
1 cup frozen peas and carrots

* See *Tips* section
** See *Measuring Pasta* section

Cookware and Utensils

12-inch skillet with lid
Small bowl

Instructions

1. Add the ground beef or ground turkey to the skillet, breaking it into small chunks, about 3/4-inch in size. Cover the skillet with the lid. Brown the ground beef or turkey on medium heat.

2. While the ground beef or turkey is browning chop the onion and the bell pepper. Add the onion and the bell pepper to the ground beef or turkey. Stir to combine.

3. Measure the sugar, salt, black pepper, garlic, caraway seed, and sweet paprika into a small bowl. Stir to combine.

4. Check the ground beef for doneness. The ground beef is fully cooked when there is no pink color. (Ground turkey is fully cooked when it is opaque.) Drain the fat if desired (this step is not necessary if ground turkey is substituted or a low-fat ground beef is used).

5. Sprinkle the seasonings over the ground beef mixture. Stir to coat the ground beef with the seasonings.

6. Add the tomato sauce to the ground beef mixture. Stir to combine.

7. Add the beef broth and the bay leaf to the ground beef and tomato mixture. Stir to combine.

8. Add the gluten-free pasta to the ground beef and tomato mixture. Stir to combine. Cover the skillet with the lid. Increase the heat to medium high until the mixture boils then reduce the heat to a gentle simmer.

9. Most gluten-free pastas cook in 7 to 12 minutes. Stir the mixture frequently, checking every 3 to 4 minutes until the pasta is cooked to your taste.

10. When the pasta is cooked to the desired doneness stir in the frozen vegetables. Cover the skillet with the lid and heat for a few minutes to thaw the vegetables. Stir again to combine. Remove the bay leaf. Serve immediately.

The Original Hamburger Macaroni Skillet

Many of us grew up enjoying the popular boxed dinners that helped busy cooks transform a pound of hamburger into a satisfying and tasty meal. Like the popular boxed dinner this hamburger and macaroni skillet is quick, convenient, and delicious.

Ingredients

1 lb ground beef or ground turkey *
1/2 cup onion, chopped
1 tsp sugar
1 tsp salt
1 tsp oregano, dried
2 tsp dried parsley flakes
1 tsp granulated garlic *
1 tsp paprika
1 tsp chili powder *
2 cups water, heated
1 cup milk *
8 oz gluten-free pasta **
2 cups shredded Cheddar cheese *
  (about 8 oz by weight)
1 cup frozen cut green beans

* See *Tips* section
** See *Measuring Pasta* section

Cookware and Utensils

12-inch skillet with lid
Small bowl
Microwave-safe liquid measuring cup
  (2-cup size or larger)
Shredder/grater
  (if not using pre-shredded cheese)

Instructions

1. Add the ground beef or ground turkey to the skillet, breaking it into small chunks, about 3/4-inch in size. Cover the skillet with the lid. Brown the ground beef or turkey on medium heat.

2. While the ground beef or turkey is browning chop the onion. Add the chopped onion to the ground beef or turkey. Stir to combine.

3. Measure the sugar, salt, oregano, parsley, garlic, paprika, and chili powder into a small bowl. Stir to combine.

4. Microwave 2 cups of water on high power for 2 minutes.

5. Check the ground beef for doneness. The ground beef is fully cooked when there is no pink color. (Ground turkey is fully cooked when it is opaque.) Drain the fat if desired (this step is not necessary if ground turkey is substituted or a low-fat ground beef is used). Sprinkle the seasonings over the cooked ground beef or turkey. Stir to coat the ground beef or turkey with the seasonings.

6. Add the hot water and the milk to the ground beef mixture. Stir to combine.

7. Add the gluten-free pasta to the ground beef mixture. Stir to combine. Cover the skillet with the lid. Increase the heat to medium high until the mixture boils then reduce the heat to a gentle simmer.

8. Most gluten-free pastas cook in 7 to 12 minutes. Stir the mixture frequently, checking every 3 to 4 minutes until the pasta is cooked to your taste.

9. While the pasta is cooking shred the Cheddar cheese (if not using pre-shredded cheese).

10. When the pasta is cooked to the desired doneness stir in the frozen green beans. Cover the skillet with the lid and heat for a few minutes to thaw the frozen green beans.

11. Add the shredded cheese to the skillet. Stir to combine. Turn off the heat and cover the skillet with the lid. When the cheese is fully melted stir again to combine. Serve immediately.

Greek Skillet with Olives and Feta

This Greek-inspired skillet is an easier version of Pastitsio, the Greek casserole of lamb, pasta, and tomatoes that is blanketed with a layer of béchamel sauce. This easier version substitutes ground beef for lamb and feta cheese for the time-consuming béchamel sauce but still retains the savory Mediterranean flavor of the original.

Ingredients

1 lb ground beef
1 cup onion, chopped
   (about 1/2 of a large onion)
1/4 tsp cinnamon
1/4 tsp black pepper
3/4 tsp salt
1/2 tsp granulated garlic *
1 tsp oregano, dried
1 cup water, heated
1 28-oz can diced tomatoes
   (do not drain)
1/2 cup red wine (substitute water)
8 oz gluten-free pasta **
4 oz feta cheese, crumbled
1 2.25-oz can sliced black olives,
   drained

* See **Tips** section
** See **Measuring Pasta** section

Cookware and Utensils

12-inch skillet with lid
Small bowl
Microwave-safe liquid measuring cup
   (1-cup size or larger)
Colander

Instructions

1. Add the ground beef to the skillet, breaking it into small chunks, about 3/4-inch in size. Cover the skillet with the lid. Brown the ground beef on medium heat.

2. While the ground beef is browning chop the onion. Add the onion to the ground beef. Stir to combine.

3. Measure the cinnamon, black pepper, salt, garlic, and oregano into a small bowl. Stir to combine.

4. Microwave 1 cup of water on high power for one minute.

5. Check the ground beef for doneness. The ground beef is fully cooked when there is no pink color. Drain the fat if desired (this step is not necessary if a low-fat ground beef is used).

6. Sprinkle the seasonings over the ground beef mixture. Stir to coat the ground beef with the seasonings.

7. Add the tomatoes (do not drain), the wine (substitute water), and the hot water to the ground beef mixture. Stir to combine.

8. Add the gluten-free pasta to the ground beef mixture. Stir to combine. Cover the skillet with the lid. Increase the heat to medium high until the mixture boils then reduce the heat to a gentle simmer.

9. Most gluten-free pastas cook in 7 to 12 minutes. Stir the mixture frequently, checking every 3 to 4 minutes until the pasta is cooked to your taste.

10. While the pasta is cooking crumble the feta cheese into a small bowl. Rinse and drain the sliced olives.

11. When the pasta is cooked to the desired doneness add the sliced olives to the skillet. Stir to combine.

12. Sprinkle the crumbled feta cheese over the skillet. Serve immediately.

Salisbury Beef and Mushroom Skillet

Salisbury steak recipes traditionally use Worcestershire sauce which often contains wheat. This Salisbury-flavored skillet substitutes wheat-free Tamari Sauce which is an earthier, richer-flavored type of soy sauce. An abundance of meaty mushrooms rounds out this savory skillet.

Ingredients

1 lb ground beef
1 cup onion, chopped
  (about 1/2 of a large onion)
8 oz white button mushrooms,
  washed and sliced
1 tsp sugar
1 tsp salt
1 tsp granulated garlic *
1/2 tsp thyme, dried
1/2 tsp black pepper
2 1/2 cups gluten-free beef broth *
1 TBSP + 1 tsp wheat-free
  Tamari Sauce *
8 oz gluten-free pasta **
1 1/2 cups frozen cut green beans

* See *Tips* section
** See *Measuring Pasta* section

Cookware and Utensils

12-inch skillet with lid
Colander
Small bowl

Instructions

1. Add the ground beef to the skillet, breaking it into small chunks, about 3/4-inch in size. Cover the skillet with the lid. Brown the ground beef on medium heat.

2. While the ground beef is browning chop the onion. Add the onion to the ground beef. Stir to combine.

3. Rinse the mushrooms in the colander and allow them to drain. Slice the mushrooms. Add the sliced mushrooms to the ground beef, stirring to combine. Cover the skillet with the lid and continue to cook on medium heat until the mushrooms are soft.

4. Measure the sugar, salt, garlic, thyme, and black pepper into a small bowl. Stir to combine.

5. Check the ground beef for doneness. The ground beef is fully cooked when there is no pink color.

6. Drain the fat if desired. This step is not necessary if a low-fat ground beef is used.

7. Sprinkle the seasonings over the beef and mushroom mixture. Stir to coat the ground beef with the seasonings.

8. Add the beef broth and 1 tablespoon plus 1 teaspoon of Tamari Sauce to the ground beef mixture. Stir to combine.

9. Add the gluten-free pasta to the ground beef mixture. Stir to combine. Cover the skillet with the lid. Increase the heat to medium high until the mixture boils then reduce the heat to a gentle simmer.

10. Most gluten-free pastas cook in 7 to 12 minutes. Stir the mixture frequently, checking every 3 to 4 minutes until the pasta is cooked to your taste.

11. When the pasta is cooked to the desired doneness stir in the frozen green beans. Cover the skillet with the lid and heat for a few minutes until the green beans are tender crisp. Stir again to combine. Serve immediately.

Mexican Beef and Rice Skillet

This Burrito in a Skillet is made with prepared salsa which cuts down on the preparation time. Choose the heat of the salsa to your taste (mild, medium, or hot).

Ingredients

1 lb ground beef
1 cup onion chopped
  (about 1/2 of a large onion)
1 green bell pepper,
  seeded and diced into 1/2" pieces
1 tsp oregano, dried
1 tsp ground cumin
1/2 tsp salt
1 24-oz jar tomato salsa (red salsa)
1 1/2 cups water, heated
1 1/2 cups converted (parboiled) rice **
2 cups shredded Cheddar cheese *
  (about 8 oz measured by weight)
1/2 cup sour cream *

* See **Tips** section
** See **Converted Rice** section

Cookware and Utensils

12-inch skillet with lid
Microwave-safe liquid measuring cup
  (2-cup size or larger)
Shredder/grater
  (if not using pre-shredded cheese)

Instructions

1. Add the ground beef to the skillet, breaking it into small chunks, about 3/4-inch in size. Cover the skillet with the lid. Brown the ground beef on medium heat.

2. While the ground beef is browning chop the onion and the bell pepper. Add the chopped onion and bell pepper to the ground beef. Stir to combine.

3. Check the ground beef for doneness. The ground beef is fully cooked when there is no pink color. Drain the fat if desired (this step is not necessary if a low-fat ground beef is used).

4. Add the oregano, cumin, and salt to the ground beef mixture. Stir to combine.

5. Add the prepared salsa to the ground beef mixture. Stir to combine.

6. Microwave 1 1/2 cups of water on high power for two minutes. Add the hot water to the ground beef mixture. Stir to combine.

7. Add the converted (parboiled) rice to the ground beef mixture. Stir to combine. Cover the skillet with the lid. Increase the heat to medium high until the mixture boils then reduce the heat to a gentle simmer. Stir occasionally.

8. While the rice is cooking shred the Cheddar cheese (if not using pre-shredded cheese).

9. When the rice is soft and the water is fully absorbed sprinkle the shredded cheese over the top of the skillet. Cover the skillet with the lid and turn off the heat. Allow the cheese to fully melt. Stir to combine the melted cheese into the rice.

10. Add the sour cream to the skillet. Stir to combine. Serve immediately.

Cheeseburger Macaroni Skillet

Who doesn't love a cheeseburger? This mouthwatering Cheeseburger in a Skillet is loaded with ground beef, red onion, and real Cheddar cheese.

Ingredients

1 lb ground beef
1/2 cup red onion, chopped
1 tsp sugar
1 1/2 tsp salt
2 tsp paprika
1 tsp chili powder *
1 tsp granulated garlic *
1/4 tsp black pepper
1 cup water, heated
1 1/2 cups milk *
8 oz gluten-free pasta **
2 cups shredded Cheddar cheese *
  (about 8 oz measured by weight)
1 cup frozen peas and carrots

* See *Tips* section
** See *Measuring Pasta* section

Cookware and Utensils

12-inch skillet with lid
Small bowl
Microwave-safe liquid measuring cup
  (1-cup size or larger)
Shredder/grater
  (if not using pre-shredded cheese)

Instructions

1. Add the ground beef to the skillet, breaking it into small chunks, about 3/4-inch in size. Cover the skillet with the lid. Brown the ground beef on medium heat.

2. While the ground beef is browning chop the onion. Add the chopped onion to the ground beef. Stir to combine.

3. Measure the sugar, salt, paprika, chili powder, garlic, and black pepper into a small bowl. Stir to combine.

4. Microwave 1 cup of water on high power for 1 minute.

5. Check the ground beef for doneness. The ground beef is fully cooked when there is no pink color. Drain the fat if desired (this step is not necessary if a low-fat ground beef is used).

6. Sprinkle the seasonings over the cooked ground beef. Stir to coat the ground beef with the seasonings.

7. Add the hot water and the milk to the ground beef mixture. Stir to combine.

8. Add the gluten-free pasta to the ground beef mixture. Stir to combine. Cover the skillet with the lid. Increase the heat to medium high until the mixture boils then reduce the heat to a gentle simmer.

9. Most gluten-free pastas cook in 7 to 12 minutes. Stir the mixture frequently, checking every 3 to 4 minutes until the pasta is cooked to your taste.

10. While the pasta is cooking shred the Cheddar cheese (if not using pre-shredded cheese).

11. When the pasta is cooked to the desired doneness stir in the frozen peas and carrots. Cover the skillet with the lid and heat for a few minutes to thaw the vegetables.

12. Add the shredded cheese to the skillet. Stir to combine. Cover the skillet with the lid and turn off the heat. Allow the cheese to fully melt. Stir again to combine the cheese. Serve immediately.

Beef & Lamb

Beef Stew in a Skillet

This skillet evokes Sunday Dinner at Grandma's house where a hearty beef stew slow-simmered for hours until the mouthwatering aroma filled the kitchen. On the days when you don't have several hours to prepare dinner this skillet offers a quick and flavorful substitute.

Ingredients

1 lb stew beef, cut into 1" cubes
2 TBSP vegetable oil
1 1/2 cups onion, sliced into crescents (about 1/2 of a large onion)
8 oz white button mushrooms, washed and sliced
1 tsp salt
1 tsp marjoram, dried
1 1/2 tsp granulated garlic *
3/4 tsp thyme, dried
1/4 tsp black pepper
1/2 cup red wine (substitute water)
2 cups gluten-free beef broth *
8 oz gluten-free pasta **
2 cups sliced frozen carrots

* See *Tips* section
** See *Measuring Pasta* section

Cookware and Utensils

12-inch skillet with lid
Colander
Small bowl

Instructions

1. Cut the beef into 1-inch cubes.

2. Add the beef and the vegetable oil to the skillet. Stir to combine. Brown the beef on medium heat.

3. While the beef is browning slice the onion into crescents. Add the onion to the beef. Stir to combine.

4. Rinse the mushrooms in the colander and allow them to drain. Slice the mushrooms. Add the sliced mushrooms to the beef and onion mixture. Stir to combine. Cover the skillet with the lid and continue to cook on medium heat until the mushrooms are soft.

5. Measure the salt, marjoram, garlic, thyme, and black pepper into a small bowl. Stir to combine.

6. When the mushrooms are soft sprinkle the seasonings over the beef and mushroom mixture. Stir to coat the beef and mushrooms with the seasonings.

7. Add the red wine (substitute water) and the beef broth to the skillet. Stir to combine.

8. Add the gluten-free pasta to the skillet. Stir to combine. Cover the skillet with the lid. Increase the heat to medium high until the mixture boils then reduce the heat to a gentle simmer.

9. Most gluten-free pastas cook in 7 to 12 minutes. Stir the mixture frequently, checking every 3 to 4 minutes until the pasta is cooked to your taste.

10. When the pasta is cooked to the desired doneness stir in the sliced frozen carrots. Cover the skillet with the lid and heat for a few minutes until the carrots are tender crisp. Serve immediately.

Stroganoff Mushroom Skillet

This savory skillet is loaded with mushrooms and gets its creamy texture from real sour cream. Lots of garlic, herbs, and spices distinguish it from the traditional flavorless stroganoff recipes. For a lower-calorie version of this dish substitute ground turkey for ground beef in the recipe.

Ingredients

1 lb ground beef or ground turkey *
1 cup onion, chopped
  (about 1/2 of a large onion)
8 oz white button mushrooms,
  washed and sliced
2 tsp salt
1 tsp sugar
2 tsp granulated garlic *
2 tsp dried parsley flakes
1/2 tsp paprika
1/4 tsp thyme, dried
1/4 tsp black pepper
1 cup water, heated
2 cups milk *
8 oz gluten-free pasta **
1 cup frozen cut green beans
1/2 cup sour cream *

* See *Tips* section
** See *Measuring Pasta* section

Cookware and Utensils

12-inch skillet with lid
Colander
Small bowl
Microwave-safe liquid measuring cup
  (1-cup size or larger)

Instructions

1. Add the ground beef or ground turkey to the skillet, breaking it into small chunks, about 3/4-inch in size. Cover the skillet with the lid. Brown the ground beef or turkey on medium heat.

2. While the ground beef or turkey is browning chop the onion. Add the onion to the ground beef or turkey. Stir to combine.

3. Rinse the mushrooms in the colander and allow them to drain. Slice the mushrooms. Add the sliced mushrooms to the ground beef or turkey, stirring to combine. Cover the skillet with the lid and continue to cook on medium heat until the mushrooms are soft.

4. Measure the salt, sugar, garlic, parsley, paprika, thyme, and black pepper into a small bowl. Stir to combine.

5. Check the ground beef for doneness. The ground beef is fully cooked when there is no pink color. (Ground turkey is fully cooked when it is opaque.) Drain the fat if desired. This step is not necessary if ground turkey is substituted or a low-fat ground beef is used. Sprinkle the seasonings over the beef and mushroom mixture. Stir to coat the ground beef and mushrooms with the seasonings.

6. Microwave 1 cup of water on high power for one minute.

7. Add the hot water and the milk to the ground beef mixture. Stir to combine.

8. Add the gluten-free pasta to the ground beef mixture. Stir to combine. Cover the skillet with the lid. Increase the heat to medium high until the mixture boils then reduce the heat to a gentle simmer. Most gluten-free pastas cook in 7 to 12 minutes. Stir the mixture frequently, checking every 3 to 4 minutes until the pasta is cooked to your taste.

9. When the pasta is cooked to the desired doneness stir in the frozen green beans. Cover the skillet with the lid and heat for a few minutes until the green beans are tender crisp.

10. Add the sour cream to the skillet. Stir to combine. Serve immediately.

Skillet Shepherd's Pie

Shepherd's Pie, also known as Cottage Pie when the recipe is made with beef instead of the traditional lamb, was a dish favored by the British working class who tended to live, not uncoincidentally, in cottages. To make this humble comfort food frugal cooks used up tidbits of meat, odds and ends of vegetables, and herbs such as rosemary, marjoram, and thyme to make a meat filling that was covered with mashed potatoes. Our easy skillet version of this traditional British dish is quicker and just as delicious.

Ingredients

For the meat filling:
10 to 12 oz frozen peas and carrots
1 lb lean ground beef
1 cup onion, chopped
  (about 1/2 of a large onion)
1 1/4 tsp salt
1/4 tsp black pepper
1/2 tsp marjoram, dried
1/4 tsp thyme, dried
1/2 tsp rosemary, dried
1 1/2 tsp granulated garlic *
1 8-oz can tomato sauce
1/2 cup red wine (substitute water)
1/4 cup water
1 TBSP cornstarch

For the mashed potato topping:
2 cups water
1 cup milk *
3 TBSP butter
3/4 tsp salt
2 1/4 cups mashed potato flakes

* See *Tips* section

Instructions

1. Transfer the frozen peas and carrots to the countertop to thaw while you prepare the ground beef filling.

2. Add the ground beef to the skillet, breaking it into small chunks, about 1/2-inch in size. Brown the ground beef on medium heat. Stir occasionally.

3. While the ground beef is browning chop the onion.

4. When the ground beef is done cooking (no pink color) drain any excess grease by moving the skillet to an unheated burner, tipping the pan away from you, and carefully spooning the excess grease into the small heatproof bowl. Allow the grease to cool before disposing. Return the skillet to the heated burner. Add the onion to the skillet. Stir to combine. Continue cooking on medium heat until the onion is soft.

5. When the onion is soft add the salt, pepper, marjoram, thyme, rosemary, and garlic to the skillet. Stir to coat the beef and onion mixture with the seasonings.

6. Add the tomato sauce, red wine (substitute water), and 1/4 cup of water to the skillet. Stir to combine.

7. Sprinkle the cornstarch over the ground beef mixture. Stir to coat the ground beef with the cornstarch to form a gravy. Cover the skillet with the lid. Reduce the heat to medium low and continue cooking until the gravy thickens.

8. When the gravy has thickened add the frozen peas and carrots to the skillet. Stir to combine. Cover the skillet with the lid. Continue cooking the beef mixture on medium low heat while you prepare the mashed potato topping.

9. Make the mashed potato topping. Add the water, milk, butter, and salt to the microwave safe mixing bowl. Microwave on high power for 3 minutes. Stir to combine the melted butter into the liquid.

Continued

Skillet Shepherd's Pie
- Continued -

Cookware and Utensils

12-inch skillet with lid
Small heatproof bowl
2-quart microwave-safe medium mixing bowl
4 wide and shallow serving bowls
Serving spoon

Instructions - continued

10. Add the mashed potato flakes to the mixing bowl. Stir to moisten the flakes. Cover the bowl with a clean paper towel to reduce splatter in the microwave. Microwave the mashed potatoes on high power for an additional 2 minutes. Stir again to completely break up the mashed potato flakes.

11. Divide the beef mixture between the serving bowls. Use a spatula to level the surface of the beef mixture in each bowl.

12. Rinse and dry the serving spoon to clean it. Use the clean serving spoon to evenly spoon the mashed potatoes over the serving bowls. Without disturbing the beef mixture use the back of the serving spoon to gently spread the mashed potatoes in an even layer over the beef mixture. Serve immediately.

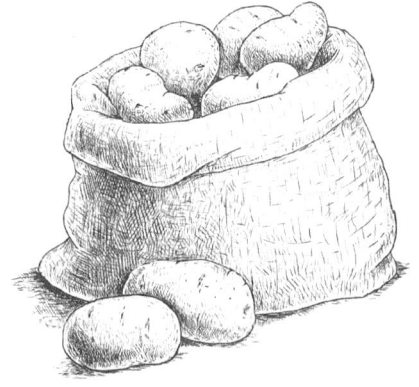

Skillet Tamale Pie

Tamale Pie is a classic comfort food of the American Southwest. Prepared with a cornmeal crust over a meat filling, its flavors mimic traditional Mexican tamales without all the work associated with making tamales. Our easy stovetop recipe uses prepared salsa and canned jalapeno peppers for convenience. To further simplify this dish the cornmeal crust is cooked on the stovetop instead of in the oven and finished with a delicious layer of melted Cheddar cheese.

Ingredients

For the filling:

1 lb lean ground beef or ground turkey *
1 4-oz can diced jalapeno peppers
  (do not drain)
1 16-oz jar red tomato salsa
  (mild, medium, or hot)
1/4 tsp salt
1 tsp oregano, dried
1 tsp granulated garlic *
2 tsp ground cumin
2 TBSP dried onion flakes
1 15-oz can black beans,
  rinsed and drained

For the topping:

1 1/4 cups cornmeal
2/3 cup gluten-free baking mix
  or gluten-free flour blend
1 TBSP sugar
1/4 tsp cayenne pepper
1/2 tsp ground cumin
1 1/2 tsp baking powder
  (do not use baking soda)
1/2 tsp salt
1 cup milk *
2 TBSP vegetable oil
1 large egg
2 cups shredded Cheddar cheese *
  (about 8 oz by weight)

* See *Tips* section

Optional Garnish:

A second 16-oz jar of red tomato salsa
(mild, medium, or hot)

Instructions

1. Add the ground beef to the skillet, breaking it into small chunks, about 1/2-inch in size. Brown the ground beef on medium heat. Stir occasionally.

2. When the ground beef is done cooking (no pink color) drain excess grease if necessary by moving the skillet to an unused burner, tipping it away from you, and spooning the excess grease into a small heatproof bowl. Allow the grease to cool before disposing. (This step is not necessary if ground turkey or a lean ground beef is used.)

3. Return the skillet to the heated burner. Add the diced jalapeno peppers (do not drain) and the salsa to the skillet. Stir to combine.

4. Add the salt, oregano, garlic, cumin, and onion to the skillet. Stir to combine.

5. Rinse the black beans in the colander and allow them to drain thoroughly. When the black beans are well drained add them to the skillet. Stir to combine.

6. Leave the skillet uncovered and allow the beef filling to simmer and reduce its liquid while you prepare the cornmeal topping. Stir occasionally.

7. Measure the cornmeal, gluten-free baking mix or gluten-free flour, sugar, cayenne pepper, and cumin into the 1-quart liquid measuring cup or medium mixing bowl. Mix well.

8. Measure the baking powder and the salt into the cornmeal mixture. Scoop the cornmeal mixture from the bottom to the top of the mixing container, mixing in a circular motion to disperse the baking powder and salt evenly throughout the cornmeal mixture.

9. Measure the milk and the vegetable oil into the 2-cup liquid measuring cup. Break the egg into the milk and oil mixture. Discard the egg shell. Puncture the egg yolk with the tines of a fork. Using the fork as a whisk stir briskly to blend the oil, egg, and milk.

Continued

Skillet Tamale Pie
- Continued -

Cookware and Utensils

12-inch skillet with lid
Colander
Small heatproof bowl
1-quart liquid measuring cup
  or medium mixing bowl
2-cup liquid measuring cup (or larger)
Scraper spatula to spread
  cornmeal topping
Shredder/grater
  (if not using pre-shredded cheese)
Wide spatula for serving

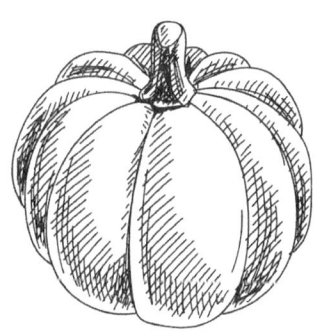

Instructions - continued

10. Pour the milk and egg mixture into the cornmeal mixture. Stir well to combine, breaking up any lumps by pressing them against the side of the mixing container with the back of the mixing spoon.

11. When the liquid in the ground beef filling has reduced to a thick sauce use the back side of a spoon to level the ground beef mixture in the skillet.

12. Use a clean spatula to spread the cornmeal batter over the top of the ground beef mixture, taking care not to disturb the meat filling under the topping.

13. Cover the skillet with the lid. Adjust the heat to medium low to gently simmer for 10 minutes. Do not uncover the skillet while the cornmeal crust is cooking.

14. While the cornmeal crust is cooking grate the Cheddar cheese (if not using pre-grated cheese).

15. After 10 minutes of cooking time test the cornmeal crust for doneness. Insert the tines of a fork into the cornmeal crust. Withdraw the utensil and examine for wetness. If no wet batter clings to the utensil then the cornmeal crust is done cooking. Continue cooking, covered, if necessary until the cornmeal is fully cooked.

16. When the cornmeal is fully cooked sprinkle the shredded Cheddar cheese evenly over the cornmeal crust. Cover the skillet with the lid, turn off the heat, and allow the cheese to melt. Let the tamale pie rest for at least 5 minutes to make it easier to portion a serving.

17. When the tamale pie has rested for 5 minutes serve by using a wide spatula to section the pie into wedges. Top with additional salsa if desired.

Savory Beef Stew with Winter Vegetables

In old fashioned days Sunday Dinner meant Grandma's Beef Stew slow-simmered all afternoon until it filled the kitchen with the mouthwatering fragrance of savory onions, flavorful herbs, and fork-tender beef. This version of Grandma's classic recipe is perfect for a Sunday Dinner when you have a little extra time to slow simmer the beef to falling apart tenderness. Warm some gluten-free bread spread with a generous serving of butter to sop up every last drop of this hearty, flavorful stew.

Ingredients

1 1/2 lbs stew beef or beef chuck roast, cut into 3/4" cubes
2 TBSP vegetable oil
1 large onion, sliced into crescents
6 carrots, scrubbed and cut into 1" lengths
3 large potatoes, scrubbed and cut into 1" cubes
2 tsp salt
1/2 tsp black pepper
1 tsp marjoram, dried
1/2 tsp oregano, dried
3/4 tsp thyme, dried
1 quart gluten-free beef broth * (reserve 1 cup)
1 cup red wine (substitute water)
1 8-oz can tomato sauce
1/4 cup cornstarch
1 cup frozen peas (optional)

* See *Tips* section

Optional Warm Bread and Butter

8 slices gluten-free bread
3 TBSP butter

Cookware and Utensils

6-quart stockpot with lid
Liquid measuring cup (2-cup size or larger)
Aluminum foil (optional)

Instructions

1. If you will be serving the (optional) warm buttered gluten-free bread then preheat the oven to 200 degrees F. Butter slices of gluten-free bread on one side. Assemble the slices into a loaf and wrap the loaf in aluminum foil. Warm the wrapped loaf in the oven while you are preparing the stew.

2. Cut the beef into 3/4-inch cubes. Add the beef and the oil to the stockpot. Stir to coat the beef with the oil. Brown the beef on medium heat, turning to brown the beef on all sides.

3. While the beef is browning slice the onion into crescents. Scrub the carrots under running water and trim their ends. Cut the carrots into 1-inch lengths. Scrub the potatoes under running water. Cut the potatoes into 1-inch cubes.

4. After the beef has browned add the onion to the stockpot. Stir to combine. Continue cooking on medium heat, stirring occasionally, until the onion is soft.

5. When the onion is soft add the salt, pepper, marjoram, oregano, and thyme to the stockpot. Stir to coat the beef and onion mixture with the seasonings. Add the potatoes and carrots to the stockpot. Stir to combine.

6. Add 3 cups of the beef broth, the red wine (substitute water), and the tomato sauce to the stockpot. Stir to combine.

7. Transfer the remaining cup of beef broth into the liquid measuring cup. Add the cornstarch to the measuring cup. Stir the broth with a fork to dissolve the cornstarch. Add the beef broth and cornstarch mixture to the stockpot.

8. Stir the stew continuously for a minute or two until it thickens. When the stew has thickened adjust the heat until the stew simmers gently. Cover the stockpot with the lid and simmer, stirring occasionally, until the beef is tender and the carrots and potatoes pierce easily with the tines of a fork.

9. When the vegetables are tender add the (optional) frozen peas. Stir to combine. Continue simmering for a minute or two to thaw the peas.

10. Serve the stew hot with (optional) warm buttered gluten-free bread.

Classic Beef Chili

This Classic Beef Chili is made with ground beef, red kidney beans, and tomatoes. I like to call this Weeknight Chili because it is a quick and easy one-pot meal for those days when you don't have a lot of time to cook dinner. This chili pairs well with our Gluten-Free Cornbread Muffin recipe.

Ingredients

1 1/2 lbs ground beef
1 large onion, chopped
4 ribs celery,
  sliced into 3/8" thick slices
2 TBSP + 1 tsp chili powder *
1 1/4 tsp ground cumin
1 1/2 tsp granulated garlic *
1 tsp oregano, dried
1 tsp salt
1/2 tsp sugar
1/4 tsp black pepper
1/4 tsp cayenne pepper
1 28-oz can tomatoes, crushed or diced
  (do not drain)
1 8-oz can tomato sauce
1 15-oz can red kidney beans,
  rinsed and drained
Optional Garnish
1 cup shredded Cheddar cheese *
  (about 4 oz by weight)

* See *Tips* section

Cookware and Utensils

6-quart stockpot with lid
Small bowl
Colander
Shredder/grater (optional)
  (if not using pre-shredded cheese)

Instructions

1. Add the ground beef to the stockpot, breaking it into small chunks, about 3/4-inch in size. Brown the ground beef on medium heat. Stir occasionally.

2. While the ground beef is browning chop the onion. Slice the celery into 3/8-inch thick slices.

3. When the ground beef is completely cooked (no pink color) drain the excess fat from the stockpot. This step is not necessary if a lean ground beef is used.

4. Add the onion and the celery to the stockpot. Stir to combine. Continue cooking on medium heat until the onion is soft.

5. Add the chili powder, cumin, garlic, oregano, salt, sugar, black pepper, and cayenne pepper to the small bowl. Stir to combine.

6. When the onion is soft add the mixed seasonings to the stockpot. Stir to combine.

7. Add the canned tomatoes (do not drain) and the tomato sauce to the stockpot. Stir to combine.

8. Rinse the kidney beans in the colander. Allow the beans to drain thoroughly. Add the kidney beans to the stockpot. Stir gently to combine. Increase the heat to medium high until the chili boils then reduce the heat to a gentle simmer. Simmer uncovered for 20 minutes to combine flavors. Stir occasionally.

9. If desired, shred the (optional) Cheddar cheese for a garnish. Transfer the shredded Cheddar cheese to the refrigerator until serving.

10. When the chili has simmered for 20 minutes it is done. Serve the chili hot. Top each bowl with (optional) shredded Cheddar cheese.

Gluten-Free Cornbread Muffins

These cornbread muffins pair well with our chili and stew recipes. Any commercially available gluten-free baking mix or gluten-free flour blend can be used in the recipe. For best results and to ensure a moist muffin that doesn't crumble remove the muffins when they are slightly underdone. They will continue to cook in the pan while they cool. Serve these cornbread muffins with butter and honey if desired. This recipe makes 12 muffins.

Ingredients

1 1/4 cups cornmeal
2/3 cup gluten-free baking mix
  or gluten-free flour blend
1/2 cup sugar
1 1/2 tsp baking powder
  (do not use baking soda)
1/2 tsp salt
1 1/4 cup milk *
1/3 cup vegetable oil plus additional oil
  for greasing the muffin pan
1 egg

* See *Tips* section

Optional Toppings

4 TBSP butter
4 TBSP honey

Instructions

1. Arrange the oven racks so that the muffin pan(s) can be centered in the middle of the oven. Preheat the oven to 350 degrees F. If you will be serving the muffins with butter (optional) then transfer the butter from the refrigerator to your countertop so that it can soften while you are preparing the muffins. If you will be serving the muffins with honey (optional) and you store your honey in the refrigerator then transfer it from the refrigerator to your countertop at this time also.

2. Measure the cornmeal, the gluten-free baking mix or gluten-free flour, and the sugar into the 2-quart liquid measuring cup or medium mixing bowl. Use a large-bowl spoon to evenly combine the dry ingredients.

3. Measure the baking powder and salt into the dry ingredients. Use the large-bowl spoon to scoop the dry ingredients from the bottom to the top of the mixing container. Mix in a circular motion, dispersing the baking powder and salt evenly throughout the cornmeal mixture.

4. Measure the milk and 1/3 cup of the vegetable oil into the 2-cup liquid measuring cup. Break the egg into the milk and oil mixture. Discard the egg shell. Puncture the egg yolk with the tines of a fork. Using the fork as a whisk stir briskly to blend the oil, egg, and milk.

5. Slowly pour the liquid ingredients into the dry ingredients. Stir well to combine the liquid and dry ingredients. Break up any lumps by pressing them against the mixing container with the back of the spoon. The batter will be thin.

6. Use a clean paper towel wetted with a few tablespoons of vegetable oil to oil the bottom and sides of the muffin pan wells. You may also use paper or foil muffin pan liners.

7. Pour or spoon the muffin batter into the oiled wells of the muffin pan. Fill each muffin well approximately 3/4 full with batter.

Continued

Gluten-Free Cornbread Muffins

- Continued -

Cookware and Utensils

2-quart liquid measuring cup
  or medium mixing bowl
Plastic or metal large-bowl spoon
2-cup liquid measuring cup (or larger)
Paper towels
Muffin pan(s)
Cooling rack (optional)

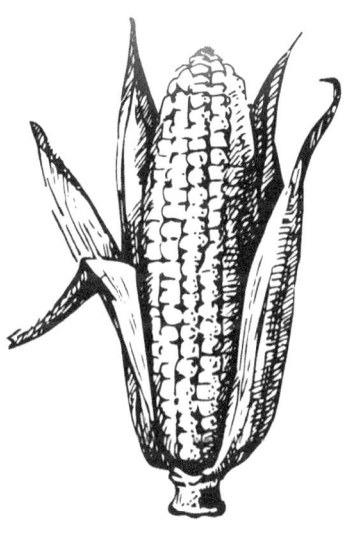

Instructions - continued

8. Transfer the muffin pan to the middle rack of the pre-heated oven. Bake for 18 minutes at 350 degrees F.

9. After 18 minutes of baking time test the muffins for doneness. Insert a toothpick or the tines of a fork into a muffin. Withdraw the utensil and examine for wetness. If no wet batter clings to the utensil then the muffins are done. Otherwise continue to bake for 2 more minutes and test again. Repeat the process until no wet batter clings to the testing utensil. Do not overcook. Overcooking will cause the muffins to crumble after they cool. Muffins that are done may not be browned on the top.

10. When the muffins are done cooking transfer the muffin pan from the oven to a cooling rack. You may also use the raised grate of a gas stove or the unenergized burner of an electric stove instead of a cooling rack. Allow the muffins to cool until they are just barely warm. Serve the warm muffins with honey and softened butter if desired.

Easy Vegetable Beef Soup

This hearty Vegetable Beef Soup is quick and easy. It requires little tending once the ingredients have been added and is perfect for those nights when you have other tasks to complete while you're making dinner. It makes use of frozen mixed vegetables and canned tomatoes for convenience so that you can use the time you save to fold a load of laundry, help the kids with their homework, or relax and unwind after your workday.

Ingredients

10 to 12 oz frozen mixed vegetables
1 quart gluten-free beef broth *
1 tsp salt
1/2 tsp black pepper
1/4 tsp marjoram, dried
1/2 tsp oregano, dried
1/2 tsp granulated garlic *
1 bay leaf
1 1/2 lbs stew beef or beef chuck roast,
  cut into 3/4" cubes
1 cup onion, chopped
  (about 1/2 of a large onion)
1 lb potatoes, scrubbed,
  diced into 1/2" cubes
1 15-oz can tomatoes, diced or crushed
  (do not drain)

* See *Tips* section

Optional Warm Bread and Butter

8 slices gluten-free bread
3 TBSP butter

Cookware and Utensils

6-quart stockpot with lid
Aluminum foil (optional)

Instructions

1. Transfer the frozen vegetables to the countertop to allow them to thaw while you are preparing the other ingredients.

2. If you will be serving the (optional) warm buttered gluten-free bread then preheat the oven to 200 degrees F. Butter slices of gluten-free bread on one side. Assemble the slices into a loaf and wrap the loaf in aluminum foil. Warm the wrapped loaf in the oven while you are preparing the soup.

3. Add the beef broth, salt, pepper, marjoram, oregano, garlic, and the bay leaf to the stockpot. Stir to combine. Cover the stockpot with the lid. Heat on medium high heat until the broth begins to boil then reduce the heat to a gentle simmer.

4. Trim excess fat from the beef and cut it into 3/4-inch cubes. Add the beef to the stockpot. Stir to combine.

5. Chop the onion. Add the onion to the stockpot. Stir to combine.

6. Scrub the potatoes under running water and dice them into 1/2-inch cubes. Add the potatoes to the stockpot. Stir to combine.

7. Add the tomatoes to the stockpot (do not drain). Stir to combine.

8. Add the thawed vegetables to the stockpot. Stir to combine. Cover the stockpot with the lid. Increase the heat to medium high until the soup begins to boil then reduce the heat to a gentle simmer. Simmer the soup, covered, until the beef is fully cooked and the potatoes pierce easily with the tines of a fork.

9. After the potatoes are tender remove the bay leaf. Serve the soup hot with (optional) warm buttered gluten-free bread.

Saucy Cabbage and Hamburger Soup

Remember the Cabbage Soup Diet? Our version of that popular soup adds ground beef or lean ground turkey for a quick and easy one-pot meal. This soup is loaded with healthy cabbage, celery, and green pepper in a saucy tomato and beef broth. It tastes so good you won't think of cabbage soup as diet food ever again.

Ingredients

1 lb ground beef or ground turkey *
3/4 cup red onion, sliced into crescents
1 green bell pepper,
   seeded and diced into 1/2" pieces
3 ribs celery, sliced into 3/8" thick slices
1 small cabbage (about 1 1/2 lbs),
   cored and sliced into 1/2" thick strips,
   strips halved
1 quart gluten-free beef broth *
1 28-oz can tomatoes, diced or crushed
   (do not drain)
1 tsp salt
1/4 tsp black pepper
1/2 tsp oregano, dried
1/2 tsp basil, dried
1/2 tsp hot red pepper flakes
1 tsp granulated garlic *

* See **Tips** section

Cookware and Utensils

6-quart stockpot with lid

Instructions

1. Add the ground beef (substitute ground turkey) to the stockpot, breaking it into small chunks, about 3/4-inch in size. Brown the ground beef on medium heat. Stir occasionally.

2. While the ground beef is browning slice the onion into thin crescents.

3. Wash, seed, and dice the bell pepper into 1/2-inch pieces.

4. Trim the ends of the celery and slice it into thin slices, about 3/8-inch thick.

5. When the ground beef is fully cooked drain the fat if desired. (This step is not necessary if you are using a lean ground beef or substituting ground turkey.) Ground beef is fully cooked when there is no pink color. Ground turkey is fully cooked when it is opaque.

6. Add the onion, bell pepper, and celery to the stockpot. Stir to combine. Cook on medium heat, stirring occasionally, until the onion is soft.

7. While the beef and vegetables are cooking prepare the cabbage. Remove the tough outer leaves of the cabbage and discard. Cut the cabbage into quarters and carve out the tough inner core of each quarter. Discard the core material. Slice the cabbage into slices about 1/2-inch thick. Halve each slice.

8. When the onion is soft add the beef broth, tomatoes (do not drain), salt, black pepper, oregano, basil, red pepper flakes, and the garlic to the stockpot. Stir to combine. Cover the stockpot with the lid. Increase the heat to medium high until the soup boils then reduce the heat to a gentle simmer.

9. When the soup is simmering add the sliced cabbage in layers over the top of the soup. Spoon some hot liquid over the cabbage then cover the stockpot with the lid to steam the cabbage. Simmer gently until the cabbage is tender.

10. When the cabbage is tender stir the soup to distribute the cabbage evenly. Serve the soup hot.

October Cider Stew

Stewing meat in apple cider makes even the toughest cuts turn to 'falling off the bone' tender in less time because the cider contains an acid that acts as a meat tenderizer. The apple cider and apple cider vinegar used in this recipe impart a sweet and tangy taste to this classic beef stew. Feel free to use pork if it is plentiful, the result will be equally delicious.

Ingredients

1 1/2 lbs beef stew meat,
  cut into 1" cubes
  (substitute boneless pork shoulder)
1 1/2 tsp salt
1/4 tsp black pepper
1 tsp thyme, dried
3 cups apple cider or apple juice
  (reserve 1 cup)
2 TBSP apple cider vinegar
3 medium potatoes, cut into 1" cubes
6 carrots, trimmed and cut
  into 1" lengths
1 large onion, sliced into crescents
1/4 cup cornstarch

Cookware and Utensils

6-quart stockpot with lid
Liquid measuring cup or small bowl
  (2-cup size or larger)

Instructions

1. Cut the beef stew meat (substitute boneless pork shoulder) into 1-inch cubes.

2. Add the beef (or pork), salt, pepper, thyme, 2 cups of the apple cider, and the apple cider vinegar to the stockpot. Reserve the remaining cup of apple cider. Stir to combine. Cover the stockpot with the lid. Heat on medium high heat until the liquid begins to boil then reduce the heat to a gentle simmer.

3. While the meat is simmering scrub the potatoes and carrots under running water. Cut the potatoes into 1-inch cubes. Trim the ends of the carrots and cut them into 1-inch lengths.

4. Slice the onion into crescents.

5. After the meat has simmered for 30 minutes measure the reserved cup of apple cider into the liquid measuring cup. Add the cornstarch to the reserved apple cider, stirring with a fork until the cornstarch is completely dissolved into the cider. Stir the stew and slowly pour the cornstarch and cider mixture into the stockpot. Stir continuously until the stew thickens to avoid clumping of the cornstarch.

6. Add the potatoes, carrots, and onions to the stockpot. Stir to combine. Cover the stockpot with the lid. Increase the heat to medium high until the stew boils then reduce the heat to a gentle simmer.

7. Simmer the stew, stirring occasionally, until the vegetables pierce easily with the tines of a fork.

8. When the vegetables are tender the stew is done. Serve the stew hot.

Herbed French (Italian) Onion Soup

Onion Soup dates back to Roman times and is an example of the Italian style of cooking known as Cucina Povera ('poor kitchen'). This rustic and economical peasant soup was adapted by the French to give it a twist of elegance by caramelizing the onions and topping the soup with expensive French cheese. Our version harkens back to the soup's humble Italian origins by skipping the time-consuming caramelization step and topping the croutons with readily-available Swiss cheese.

Ingredients

3 TBSP butter
1 1/2 lbs yellow onions
  (about 3 large onions),
  sliced thinly into rings,
  rings sliced in half
1 1/2 tsp salt
1/4 tsp black pepper
1/2 tsp sugar
1/4 tsp thyme, dried
1/2 tsp rosemary, dried
1/4 tsp granulated garlic *
1 quart gluten-free beef broth *
1/2 cup white wine (substitute water)
1 TBSP + 2 tsp gluten-free
  Worcestershire Sauce *
2 bay leaves

For the Croutons
8 slices gluten-free bread
1 cup shredded Swiss cheese *
  (about 4 oz by weight)

* See *Tips* section

Cookware and Utensils

6-quart stockpot with lid
Metal baking sheet
Shredder/grater
  (if not using pre-shredded cheese)

Instructions

1. Preheat the oven to 300 degrees F. Add the butter to the stockpot. Melt the butter on low heat.

2. Peel the onions and slice them into thin rings. Cut the sliced rings in half to make thin crescents of onion. Add the onion crescents to the stockpot, separating them as you add them. Stir to coat the onions with the melted butter. Cover the stockpot with the lid. Increase the heat to medium and cook, stirring frequently, until the onions are soft.

3. While the onions are cooking place the slices of gluten-free bread (croutons) on the baking sheet. Transfer the baking sheet to the oven. Toast the first side of the croutons until slightly crunchy (about 10 minutes) then remove the baking sheet from the oven.

4. When the onion is soft add the salt, pepper, sugar, thyme, rosemary, and garlic to the stockpot. Stir to combine.

5. Add the beef broth, white wine (substitute water), gluten-free Worcestershire Sauce, and the bay leaves to the stockpot. Stir to combine. Cover the stockpot with the lid. Increase the heat to medium high until the soup boils then reduce the heat to a gentle simmer. Simmer for 10 minutes or more to combine flavors.

6. When the croutons are cool flip each crouton over. Return the baking sheet to the oven. Toast the croutons until their top side is just barely turning a light golden brown (about 10 minutes).

7. While the croutons are toasting shred the Swiss cheese (if not using pre-shredded cheese).

8. When the croutons are just barely browned remove the baking sheet from the oven. Sprinkle the shredded Swiss cheese over the croutons. Return the baking sheet to the oven. Bake the croutons until the cheese melts and just begins to brown then turn off the oven to keep the croutons warm until serving.

9. At serving time remove the bay leaves from the stockpot. Serve the soup hot with the warm croutons on the side.

Mediterranean Lamb Stew

This savory stew features ingredients found in traditional Mediterranean cooking: lamb, olive oil, red wine, tomatoes, and lots of herbs and garlic. Use a hearty and flavorful red wine like a Cabernet Sauvignon or Syrah to make this stew. Enjoy the rest of the bottle with dinner.

Ingredients

1 1/2 lbs boneless lamb, cut into 1" cubes
2 TBSP olive oil
1 1/2 cups onion, sliced into crescents
6 cloves garlic, chopped
3 carrots, ends trimmed
  and sliced into 1/2" thick rounds
1 1/2 lbs potatoes, cut into 1" cubes
1 1/2 tsp salt
1/2 tsp black pepper
1 tsp rosemary, dried
1/2 tsp oregano, dried
3/4 tsp thyme, dried
1/2 tsp marjoram, dried
2 cups gluten-free beef broth *
3 TBSP cornstarch
3/4 cup red wine
1 8-oz can tomato sauce
2 bay leaves

* See *Tips* section

Cookware and Utensils

6-quart stockpot with lid
Liquid measuring cup
  (2-cup size or larger)
  or medium bowl

Instructions

1. Trim excess fat from the lamb. Cut the lamb into 1-inch cubes. Add the lamb and the olive oil to the stockpot. Stir to coat the lamb with the olive oil. Brown the lamb on medium heat, turning frequently to brown all sides.

2. While the lamb is browning slice the onion into crescents. Chop the garlic.

3. When the lamb has browned add the onion and the garlic to the stockpot. Stir to combine.

4. Scrub the carrots under running water and trim their ends. Slice the carrots into 1/2-inch thick rounds. Add the carrots to the stockpot. Stir to combine.

5. Scrub the potatoes under running water. Cut the potatoes into 1-inch cubes. Add the potatoes to the stockpot. Stir to combine.

6. Add the salt, pepper, rosemary, oregano, thyme, and marjoram to the stockpot. Stir to coat the lamb and vegetables with the seasonings.

7. Measure 2 cups of beef broth into the liquid measuring cup or bowl. Add the cornstarch to the beef broth. Stir with a fork to completely dissolve the cornstarch into the broth. Slowly add the broth to the stockpot, stirring the stew continuously to avoid clumping the cornstarch.

8. Add the red wine, tomato sauce, and the bay leaves to the stockpot. Stir to combine. Cover the stockpot with the lid. Increase the heat to medium high until the stew boils then reduce the heat to a gentle simmer. Simmer the stew, covered, until the potatoes and carrots pierce easily with the tines of a fork.

9. When the vegetables are tender remove the bay leaves. Serve the stew hot.

Stuffed Pepper Soup

Making a dish of baked bell peppers stuffed with a spicy tomato, beef, and rice filling is a time-consuming process. If you like the taste of stuffed peppers you will love this soup which duplicates the taste of the traditional baked dish yet is on the table in no time.

Ingredients

1 lb ground beef
2 cups onion, chopped
  (about 1 large onion)
2 green bell peppers, seeded and
  diced into 1/2" pieces
1 1/2 tsp salt
1/2 tsp black pepper
1/2 tsp cayenne pepper
1/2 tsp oregano, dried
1 tsp granulated garlic *
1/2 tsp hot red pepper flakes
1 quart gluten-free beef broth *
1 cup water
1 cup converted (parboiled) rice **
1 TBSP brown sugar, firmly packed
1 15-oz can tomato sauce
  (substitute two 8-oz cans tomato sauce)
1 15-oz can tomatoes, diced or crushed
  (do not drain)

* See *Tips* section
** See *Converted Rice* section

Cookware and Utensils

6-quart stockpot with lid
Small heatproof bowl

Instructions

1. Add the ground beef to the skillet, breaking it into small chunks, about 3/4-inch in size. Brown the ground beef on medium heat until it is fully cooked (no pink color).

2. While the ground beef is browning chop the onion. Wash, seed, and dice the bell peppers into 1/2-inch pieces.

3. When the ground beef is fully cooked drain the grease by moving the stockpot to an unheated burner, tipping it away from you, and carefully spooning the excess grease into a small heatproof bowl. Reserve about 2 tablespoons of drippings. Allow the excess grease to cool before disposing.

4. Return the stockpot to the heated burner. Add the onion and bell pepper to the stockpot. Stir to combine. Continue cooking on medium heat until the onion is soft. Stir occasionally.

5. When the onion is soft add the salt, black pepper, cayenne pepper, oregano, garlic, and hot pepper flakes to the stockpot. Stir to combine.

6. Add the beef broth, 1 cup of water, and the converted (parboiled) rice to the stockpot. Stir to combine. Cover the stockpot with the lid. Heat the broth on medium high heat until it boils then adjust the heat to a gentle simmer. Simmer, covered, until the rice is fully cooked.

7. While the rice is cooking measure 1 tablespoon of brown sugar by firmly packing it into the measuring spoon and leveling the top. Add the brown sugar to the stockpot. Stir to combine. Continue cooking until the rice is fully cooked.

8. When the rice is fully cooked add the tomato sauce and the tomatoes (do not drain) to the stockpot. Stir to combine. Simmer the soup for 10 minutes to combine flavors. Serve immediately.

Easy Vietnamese Pho

Pho (pronounced 'fuh') is the beef-based Vietnamese equivalent of the classic American comfort food Chicken Noodle Soup. Pho is traditionally prepared by slow-simmering marrow bones and exotic spices such as star anise for hours to produce a rich beef broth that is poured over rice noodles and thinly sliced uncooked beef. As the hot broth cooks the beef to a medium rare perfection condiments such as bean sprouts, cilantro, scallions, and basil are added.

Ingredients

1 lb beef round steak, sliced across the grain into 1/4" thick slices
2 quarts gluten-free beef broth *
3/4 tsp Chinese Five Spice Powder *
1/2 tsp ground coriander
1/4 tsp ground ginger
1 lime, juiced (about 1 TBSP juice)
1 1/2 tsp dried onion flakes
1 1/2 tsp Asian chili sauce (substitute Sriracha sauce)
3 TBSP Asian fish sauce
12 to 14 oz Pad Thai-style rice noodles

* See *Tips* section

Optional Condiments

1 bunch green onions (scallions), sliced into 3/8" thick slices
1 bunch cilantro, stems removed, leaves coarsely chopped
1 handful basil leaves, sliced into ribbons
1 cup bean sprouts

Instructions

1. Transfer the beef to the freezer so that it partially freezes while you are preparing the broth. This will make it easier to slice the beef into thin slices.

2. Add the beef broth to the stockpot. Heat the broth on medium high heat until the broth boils then reduce the heat to a gentle simmer.

3. Add the Chinese Five Spice Powder, the coriander, and the ginger to the broth. Stir to combine.

4. Juice the lime into the small bowl or liquid measuring cup. Set aside the lime juice.

5. Rinse the (optional) condiments in the colander and allow them to drain thoroughly. Trim the ends of the green onions and slice them into 3/8-inch thick slices. Remove the stems from the cilantro and coarsely chop the leaves. Slice the basil leaves into thin ribbons. Rinse and drain the bean sprouts. Transfer the condiments to their own small serving bowls and refrigerate until serving time.

6. Remove the partially frozen beef from the freezer. Slice the beef thinly against the grain into 1/4-inch thick slices.

7. Transfer several pieces of the raw sliced beef into the basket of a metal mesh sieve. Slowly lower the sieve into the broth and suspend it in the broth to pre-cook the beef. Let the beef remain in the broth for a minute or two until it just barely loses its pink color (medium rare). When the beef has finished cooking lift the sieve out of the hot broth and allow it to drain over the stockpot. After the broth has drained from the beef transfer the cooked beef to the clean medium bowl. Repeat until all the beef has been pre-cooked.

8. Add the dried onion flakes, reserved lime juice, chili sauce (substitute Sriracha sauce), and the fish sauce to the broth. Stir to combine.

Continued

Easy Vietnamese Pho - continued

Pho is known for its time-consuming preparation and use of ingredients that are not commonly found outside of Asian kitchens. This version takes a shortcut by using packaged beef broth and readily-available Chinese Five Spice Powder. The beef is pre-cooked in the broth to ensure it is sufficiently cooked before serving. While this version makes no claims to be as good as traditionally prepared Pho it does satisfy when you want a quick and easy bowl of this famous Vietnamese 'comfort soup'.

Cookware and Utensils

6-quart stockpot with lid
Citrus juicer
Small bowl or liquid measuring cup
Colander
Small serving bowls for condiments
Metal mesh sieve
Medium bowl
Kitchen tongs
4 deep soup bowls
Ladle

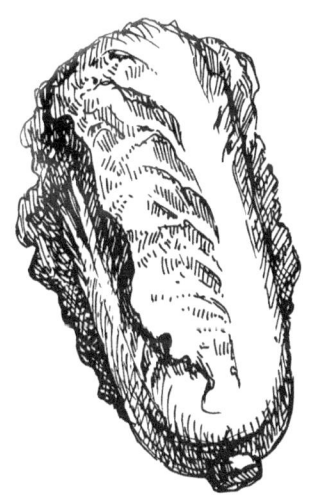

Instructions - continued

9. Add half the uncooked noodles to the simmering broth. Allow the noodles to cook in the broth until they are soft. Do not overcook.

10. When the noodles are soft use the kitchen tongs to lift the noodles out of the broth. Divide the noodles between four serving bowls.

11. Use the kitchen tongs to transfer half of the pre-cooked beef to the serving bowls. Arrange the beef on top of the noodles.

12. Add the remaining uncooked noodles to the broth. Allow the noodles to cook in the broth until they are soft.

13. When the noodles are soft use the kitchen tongs to lift the noodles out of the broth. Divide the noodles between the four serving bowls, layering them over the beef.

14. Use the kitchen tongs to transfer the remaining pre-cooked beef to the serving bowls. Arrange the beef over the top of the noodles.

15. Ladle the hot broth over the noodles and beef, dividing the broth evenly between the serving bowls.

16. Remove the condiments from the refrigerator. Serve the soup immediately. Top the soup with (optional) condiments if desired.

Hot and Smoky Beer and Bacon Chili

Chili and beer is a great combination and this chili contains everything - bacon, beef, and beer - that a chili lover could want. If you thought you had to give up beer when you went gluten-free then think again. With an ever-increasing range of gluten-free beers available, beer lovers who want to avoid gluten have choices. Use a good quality smoked paprika for this recipe - regular paprika won't do it justice.

Ingredients

6 slices bacon, diced into 1/2" pieces
1 1/2 cups red onion,
  sliced into crescents
3 cloves garlic, chopped
1 1/2 lbs lean ground beef
1 1/2 tsp ground cumin
1 1/2 tsp smoked paprika
1 tsp cayenne pepper
1 tsp salt
1 28-oz can tomatoes, diced or crushed
  (do not drain)
1/2 cup gluten-free beer
1 15-oz can red kidney beans
  or pinto beans, rinsed and drained
1 cup shredded Cheddar cheese *
  (about 4 oz by weight)

* See *Tips* section

Cookware and Utensils

6-quart stockpot with lid
Small heatproof bowl
Colander
Shredder/grater
  (if not using pre-shredded cheese)

Instructions

1. Dice the bacon into 1/2-inch pieces and add it to the stockpot. Crisp the bacon on medium heat. Stir frequently.

2. While the bacon is crisping slice the onion into crescents.

3. Chop the garlic.

4. When the bacon is crisp drain some of the grease from the stockpot by moving the stockpot to an unused burner, tipping the stockpot away from you to pool the grease, then carefully spooning the grease into a small heatproof bowl. Reserve about two tablespoons of bacon drippings in the stockpot. Allow the hot grease to cool before disposing.

5. Return the stockpot to the heated burner. Add the onion and the garlic to the stockpot. Stir to coat the onion and garlic with the bacon drippings. Cook the onion mixture on medium heat, stirring occasionally, until the onion is soft.

6. When the onion is soft add the ground beef to the stockpot, breaking it into small chunks, about 3/4-inch in size. Stir to combine. Cover the stockpot with the lid. Brown the ground beef on medium heat, stirring occasionally, until the ground beef is fully cooked (no pink color).

7. When the ground beef is fully cooked add the cumin, smoked paprika, cayenne pepper, and salt to the stockpot. Stir to combine.

8. Add the tomatoes (do not drain) and the gluten-free beer to the stockpot. Stir to combine.

9. Rinse the beans in the colander and allow them to drain thoroughly. Add the beans to the stockpot. Stir gently to combine. Cover the stockpot with the lid. Increase the heat to medium high until the chili boils then reduce the heat to a gentle simmer. Simmer the chili for 20 minutes to combine flavors.

10. While the chili is simmering shred the Cheddar cheese (if not using pre-shredded cheese).

11. After the chili has simmered for 20 minutes it is done. Serve the chili hot, topped with shredded Cheddar cheese.

Herbed Provencal Beef Stew

This hearty stew gets its origins from the slow-simmered beef daubes of Provence, a region in southern France near the Mediterranean Sea. Our version is seasoned with Herbs de Provence, a mixture of dried herbs typical of this sunny area of southern France. Herbs de Provence often includes rosemary, oregano, marjoram, thyme, savory, and lavender. If you don't have this seasoning blend in your spice cabinet then invest in a small bottle as it is an excellent seasoning for grilled or sautéed chicken.

Ingredients

3 TBSP olive oil
1 1/2 lbs stew beef or boneless chuck roast, cut into 1" cubes
1 large onion, sliced into crescents
6 cloves garlic, chopped
1 1/2 tsp salt
1/2 tsp black pepper
1 tsp thyme, dried
2 tsp Herbs de Provence, dried
1 TBSP dried parsley flakes
1/2 tsp fennel seed, slightly crushed (optional)
1 cup white wine
1 bay leaf
2 cups gluten-free beef broth *
3 TBSP cornstarch
4 carrots, ends trimmed, sliced into 1/2" thick slices
1 1/2 lbs potatoes, cut into 1" cubes

* See *Tips* section

Cookware and Utensils

6-quart stockpot with lid
Mortar and pestle or small ceramic bowl (if adding the optional crushed fennel seeds)
Liquid measuring cup (2-cup size or larger)

Instructions

1. Add the olive oil to the stockpot. Trim excess fat from the beef. Cut the beef into 1-inch cubes. Add the beef to the stockpot. Brown the beef on medium heat, stirring frequently, until all sides of the beef are browned.

2. While the beef is browning slice the onion into crescents. Chop the garlic. When the beef has browned add the onion and the garlic to the stockpot. Stir to combine. Continue cooking, stirring occasionally, until the onion is soft.

3. When the onion is soft add the salt, pepper, thyme, Herbs de Provence, and parsley to the stockpot. Stir to combine. If you will be adding the optional fennel seeds then lightly crush them with a mortar and pestle before adding them to the stockpot. If you don't have a mortar and pestle use the back side of a table spoon to crush the fennel seeds against the inside of a small ceramic bowl. You don't need to break apart the seeds into smaller pieces, just apply enough pressure to crack the tough seed coating. Lightly crushing the seeds allows their flavor to disperse more quickly into the stew.

4. Add the white wine and the bay leaf to the stockpot. Stir to combine.

5. Measure the beef broth into the liquid measuring cup. Add the cornstarch to the beef broth. Stir with a fork to completely dissolve the cornstarch into the broth. Slowly add the broth to the stockpot, stirring continuously to avoid clumping the cornstarch.

6. Scrub the carrots, trim their ends, and slice them into 1/2-inch thick rounds. Add the carrots to the stockpot. Stir to combine.

7. Scrub the potatoes and dice them into 1-inch cubes. Add the potatoes to the stockpot. Stir to combine. Cover the stockpot with the lid. Increase the heat to medium high until the stew boils then reduce the heat to a gentle simmer. Simmer the stew, stirring occasionally, until the carrots and potatoes pierce easily with the tines of a fork.

8. When the vegetables are tender remove the bay leaf. Serve the stew hot.

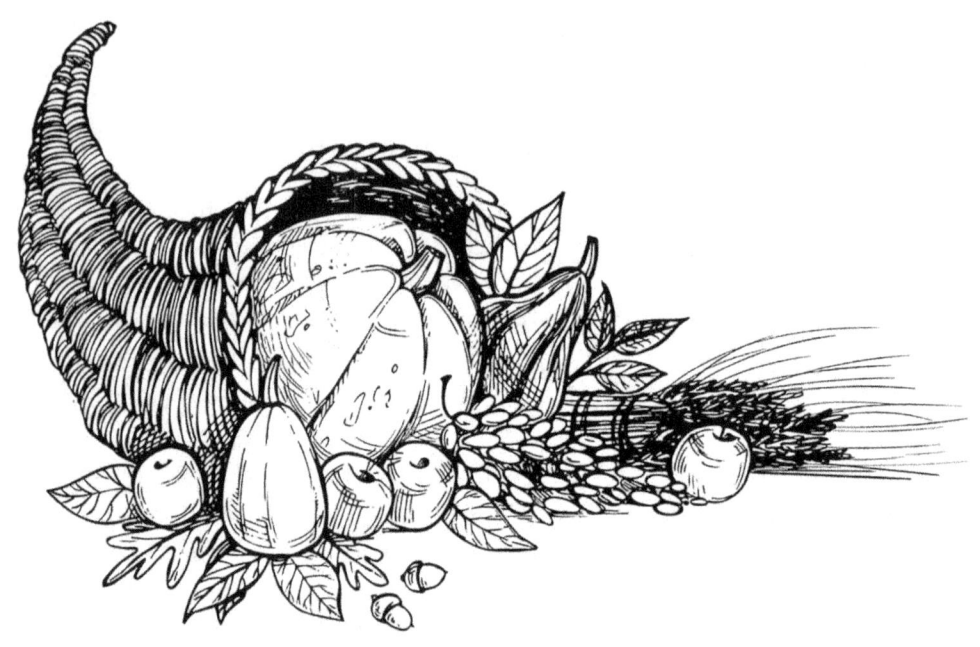

Chicken

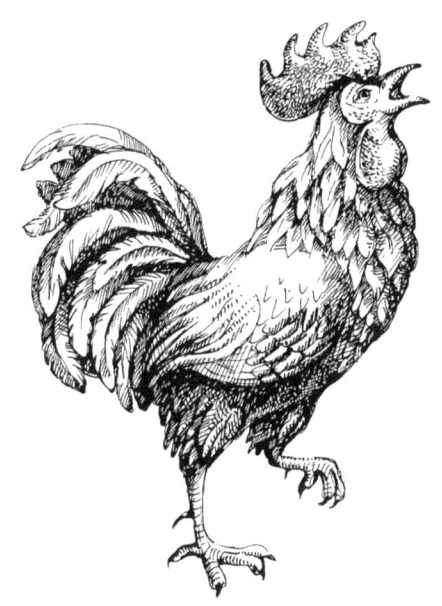

Meals in a Skillet

- 96   Southwest Fajita Skillet
- 97   Tandoori Chicken Skillet
- 98   Chicken Curry Skillet
- 99   Cheesy Chicken and Rice Skillet
- 100   Chicken Broccoli Alfredo Skillet
- 101   Stovetop Chicken Tetrazzini
- 102   Chipotle Chicken and Rice

Soups and Stews

- 104   Classic Chicken Noodle Soup
- 105   White Bean Chili with Chicken and Red Onion
- 106   California Rancho Posole
- 107   Chicken and Rice Soup
- 108   Southwestern Chicken Stew
- 110   Chicken and Vegetable Bean Soup
- 111   Santa Fe Soup
- 112   Chicken and Summer Vegetable Stew
- 114   Moroccan Chicken and Apricot Stew
- 116   Italian Hunter's Chicken
- 118   Chunky Cream of Chicken and Mushroom Soup
- 119   Jalapeno Chicken and Rice Stew

Southwest Fajita Skillet

Just like the sizzling southwestern stir fry this skillet meal features bell peppers, onions, tangy lime, and succulent chicken. Garnish with sour cream and slices of avocado if desired.

Ingredients

1 lb boneless skinless chicken breast, cut into 1" cubes
2 TBSP vegetable oil
1 1/2 cups onion, sliced into crescents (about 1/2 of a large onion)
1 green bell pepper, seeded and cut into 1/2" strips, strips halved
1 red bell pepper, seeded and cut into 1/2" strips, strips halved
2 Roma tomatoes, washed and diced into 3/8" cubes
2 limes, juiced (about 2 TBSP juice)
1/2 tsp granulated garlic *
3 TBSP taco seasoning *
3 cups gluten-free chicken broth *
1 1/2 cups converted (parboiled) rice **
1 cup shredded Cheddar or Monterey Jack cheese * (about 4 oz by weight)

* See *Tips* section
** See *Converted Rice* section

Cookware and Utensils

12-inch skillet with lid
Citrus juicer
Shredder/grater (if not using pre-shredded cheese)

Instructions

1. Cut the chicken into 1-inch cubes.

2. Add the chicken and the oil to the skillet. Stir to combine. Cover the skillet with the lid. Cook the chicken on medium heat. Stir occasionally.

3. Slice the onion into crescents.

4. Seed the bell peppers and slice them into 1/2-inch thick strips. Cut the strips in half.

5. Rinse the Roma tomatoes. Dice the Roma tomatoes into 3/8-inch cubes.

6. Juice the limes.

7. When the chicken is done cooking (opaque all the way through when cut with a knife) add the onion and the bell pepper to the skillet. Stir to combine. Stir fry for 2 minutes on medium high heat until the bell peppers are tender crisp. Stir frequently.

8. Reduce the heat to medium. Add the Roma tomatoes and the lime juice to the skillet. Stir to combine.

9. Add the granulated garlic and the taco seasoning to the skillet. Stir to incorporate the seasonings evenly into the chicken and vegetable mixture.

10. Add the chicken broth and the converted (parboiled) rice to the skillet. Stir to combine. Cover the skillet with the lid. Increase the heat to medium high until the mixture boils then reduce the heat to a gentle simmer. Stir occasionally.

11. While the rice is cooking shred the Cheddar or Monterey Jack cheese (if not using pre-shredded cheese).

12. When the rice is soft and the water is fully absorbed sprinkle the shredded cheese over the top of the skillet. Cover the skillet with the lid. Turn off the heat and allow the cheese to fully melt. Serve immediately.

Tandoori Chicken Skillet

Preparing traditional Tandoori Chicken is a time-consuming process that involves marinating the chicken overnight in a spicy lemon yogurt sauce. This skillet version features all the flavors of the traditional dish without the long preparation time.

Ingredients

1 lb boneless skinless chicken breast or thigh meat, cut into 1" cubes
2 TBSP vegetable oil
1 1/2 cups onion, sliced into crescents (about 1/2 of a large onion)
1 lemon, juiced (about 2 TBSP juice)
6 oz gluten-free unflavored yogurt *
1/2 tsp salt
1/2 tsp ground ginger
1/2 tsp turmeric
1 tsp sugar
1 tsp ground cumin
1 1/2 tsp ground coriander
1 tsp granulated garlic *
1 tsp paprika
1/4 tsp cayenne pepper
2 1/2 cups gluten-free chicken broth *
1 1/2 cups converted (parboiled) rice **
2 cups frozen sliced carrots

* See *Tips* section
** See *Converted Rice* section

Cookware and Utensils

12-inch skillet with lid
Citrus juicer
Small bowl

Instructions

1. Cut the chicken into 1-inch cubes.

2. Add the chicken and the oil to the skillet. Stir to combine. Cover the skillet with the lid. Heat on medium heat, stirring occasionally.

3. While the chicken is cooking slice the onion into crescents.

4. Juice the lemon.

5. When the chicken is done cooking (opaque all the way through when cut with a knife) add the onion to the skillet. Stir to combine. Continue cooking on medium heat until the onion is soft.

6. When the onion is soft add the lemon juice and the yogurt to the skillet. Stir to combine.

7. Measure the salt, ginger, turmeric, sugar, cumin, coriander, garlic, paprika, and cayenne pepper into a small bowl. Stir to combine. Add the seasonings to the skillet. Stir to incorporate the seasonings evenly into the yogurt.

8. Add the chicken broth to the skillet. Stir to combine.

9. Add the converted (parboiled) rice to the skillet. Stir to combine. Cover the skillet with the lid. Increase the heat to high until the mixture boils then reduce the heat to a gentle simmer. Stir occasionally.

10. When the rice is soft and the water is fully absorbed add the frozen carrots to the skillet. Stir to combine. Cover the skillet with the lid. Heat for a few minutes until the frozen carrots are tender crisp. Serve immediately.

Chicken Curry Skillet

This coconut milk-based mild curry features tender chunks of chicken, crisp bell pepper, tangy lime, and mild yellow curry powder. Add the optional cilantro for extra flavor.

Ingredients

1 lb boneless skinless chicken breast or thigh meat, cut into 1" cubes
2 TBSP vegetable oil
1 1/2 cups onion, sliced into crescents (about 1/2 of a large onion)
1 red bell pepper, seeded and cut into 1/2" strips, strips halved
2 limes, juiced (about 2 TBSP juice)
1 13.5-oz can coconut milk ***
3 TBSP brown sugar, firmly packed
1 TBSP mild yellow (sweet) curry powder *
1 tsp ground ginger
1/2 tsp salt
1/4 tsp hot red pepper flakes
1/4 tsp granulated garlic *
2 cups water, heated
1 1/2 cups converted (parboiled) rice **
1/2 cup cilantro, stems removed, leaves coarsely chopped (optional)
2 cups frozen sliced carrots

* See *Tips* section
** See *Converted Rice* section
*** Use coconut milk without gluten-containing thickeners. Guar gum does not intentionally contain gluten.

Cookware and Utensils

12-inch skillet with lid
Citrus juicer   Small bowl
Microwave-safe liquid measuring cup (2-cup size or larger)
Colander (if using the optional cilantro)

Instructions

1. Cut the chicken into 1-inch cubes.

2. Add the chicken and the oil to the skillet. Stir to combine. Cover the skillet with the lid. Cook on medium heat, stirring occasionally.

3. While the chicken is cooking slice the onion into crescents.

4. Seed the bell pepper. Slice the bell pepper into 1/2-inch thick strips. Cut the strips in half.

5. Juice the limes.

6. When the chicken is opaque all the way through when cut with a knife add the onion and the bell pepper to the skillet. Stir to combine. Stir fry for a few minutes on medium high heat until the bell pepper is tender crisp. Stir frequently.

7. Reduce the heat to medium. Vigorously shake the can of coconut milk before opening to disperse solids. Add the coconut milk and lime juice to the skillet. Stir to combine.

8. Firmly pack the brown sugar into the measuring spoon to measure it, leveling the top of the spoon.

9. Add the brown sugar, curry powder, ginger, salt, red pepper flakes, and garlic to the small bowl. Stir the seasonings to combine. Add the seasonings to the skillet. Stir to incorporate the seasonings evenly into the coconut milk.

10. Microwave 2 cups of water on high power for 2 minutes. Add the hot water to the skillet. Stir to combine.

11. Add the converted (parboiled) rice to the skillet. Stir to combine. Cover the skillet with the lid. Increase the heat to medium high until the mixture boils then reduce the heat to a gentle simmer. Stir occasionally.

12. While the rice is cooking rinse and drain the cilantro, remove the stems, and coarsely chop the cilantro leaves (optional).

13. When the rice is soft and the water is fully absorbed add the cilantro (optional) and the frozen carrots to the skillet. Stir to combine. Cover the skillet with the lid and heat for a few minutes until the carrots are tender crisp. Serve immediately.

Cheesy Chicken and Rice Skillet

This is not your mother's chicken casserole. This flavorful casserole-in-a-skillet is loaded with lean chicken and healthy broccoli. Onions, celery, and just a pat of butter add flavor not found in those calorie-laden 'open a can of cream of chicken soup' recipes. Enjoy a second helping of this healthy, 'good for you' skillet.

Ingredients

10 to 12 oz frozen chopped broccoli
3 TBSP butter
1 lb boneless skinless chicken breast
  or thigh meat, cut into 1" cubes
1 1/2 cups onion, chopped
3 ribs celery, sliced thinly into 3/8" slices
1 1/2 tsp salt
1/2 tsp thyme, dried
1/2 tsp marjoram, dried
1/2 tsp granulated garlic *
1/4 tsp black pepper
2 cups gluten-free chicken broth *
1 cup milk *
1 1/2 cups converted (parboiled) rice **
2 cups shredded Monterey Jack cheese *
  (about 8 oz measured by weight)

* See *Tips* section
** See *Converted Rice* section

Cookware and Utensils

12-inch skillet with lid
Shredder/grater
  (if not using pre-shredded cheese)

Instructions

1. Remove the frozen chopped broccoli from the freezer. Thaw it on the countertop while preparing the chicken and rice mixture.

2. Add the butter to the skillet. Melt on low heat.

3. Cut the chicken into 1-inch cubes. Add the chicken to the melted butter. Stir to combine. Cover the skillet with the lid. Increase the heat to medium. Stir occasionally.

4. While the chicken is cooking chop the onion.

5. Slice the celery thinly into 3/8-inch thick slices.

6. When the chicken is opaque all the way through when cut with a knife add the onion and the celery to the skillet. Stir to combine. Continue cooking, stirring occasionally, until the onion is soft.

7. When the onion is soft add the salt, thyme, marjoram, garlic, and black pepper to the skillet. Stir to coat the chicken and vegetable mixture with the seasonings.

8. Add the chicken broth and the milk to the skillet. Stir to combine.

9. Add the converted (parboiled) rice to the skillet. Stir to combine. Cover the skillet with the lid. Increase the heat to medium high until the mixture boils then reduce the heat to a gentle simmer. Stir occasionally.

10. While the rice is cooking shred the Monterey Jack cheese (if not using pre-shredded cheese).

11. When the rice is soft and the water is fully absorbed add the broccoli to the skillet. Stir to combine. Cover the skillet with the lid and heat for a few minutes until the broccoli is tender crisp.

12. Add the shredded cheese to the skillet. Stir to combine. Turn off the heat and cover the skillet with the lid. Allow the cheese to fully melt. Stir again to combine the cheese. Serve immediately.

Chicken Broccoli Alfredo Skillet

This creamy skillet features a classic Alfredo sauce with lots of butter, Parmesan cheese, and garlic. Meaty chunks of chicken breast and tender crisp broccoli make this classic comfort food a complete meal.

Ingredients

10 to 12 oz frozen broccoli florets
  or frozen chopped broccoli
3 TBSP butter
1 lb boneless skinless chicken breast,
  cut into 1" cubes
1 tsp salt
2 tsp dried parsley flakes
1 1/2 tsp granulated garlic *
1/4 tsp black pepper
3/4 cup water, heated
2 cups milk *
8 oz gluten-free pasta **
1 cup grated Parmesan cheese *

* See *Tips* section
** See *Measuring Pasta* section

Cookware and Utensils

12-inch skillet with lid
Small bowl
Microwave-safe liquid measuring cup
  (1-cup size or larger)
Shredder/grater
  (if not using pre-grated cheese)

Instructions

1. Remove the frozen broccoli from the freezer and thaw it on the countertop while preparing the pasta.

2. Add the butter to the skillet. Melt the butter on low heat.

3. While the butter is melting cut the chicken into 1-inch cubes.

4. Add the chicken to the melted butter. Stir to combine. Cover the skillet with the lid. Increase the heat to medium. Cook the chicken, stirring occasionally, until it is opaque all the way through when cut with a knife.

5. Measure the salt, parsley, garlic, and black pepper into a small bowl. Stir to combine.

6. Microwave 3/4 cup of water on high power for 1 minute.

7. When the chicken is fully cooked sprinkle the seasonings over the chicken. Stir to coat the chicken with the seasonings.

8. Add the hot water and the milk to the skillet. Stir to combine.

9. Add the gluten-free pasta to the skillet. Stir to combine. Cover the skillet with the lid. Increase the heat to medium high until the mixture boils then reduce the heat to a gentle simmer.

10. While the pasta is cooking grate the Parmesan cheese (if not using pre-grated cheese).

11. If necessary, defrost the broccoli further in the microwave on low power until it separates easily (about 2 minutes). Do not overcook.

12. Most gluten-free pastas cook in 7 to 12 minutes. Stir the mixture frequently, checking every 3 to 4 minutes until the water is almost all absorbed.

13. When the pasta is nearly cooked to the desired doneness (not all the water will be absorbed yet) stir in the thawed broccoli. Continue cooking on medium heat until the pasta is fully cooked and the broccoli is tender crisp.

14. Stir in the grated Parmesan cheese. Cover the skillet with the lid. Turn off the heat. Allow the cheese to fully melt. Stir again to combine the cheese thoroughly. Serve immediately.

Stovetop Chicken Tetrazzini

Our Chicken Tetrazzini recipe is derived from a dish that was created in the early 1900's for Italian opera singer Luisa Tetrazzini. An Italian coloratura soprano who worked under contract for Oscar Hammerstein, Tetrazzini was pals with Italian tenor Enrico Caruso and often sang in San Francisco. Her passion for good food was legendary, she ate spaghetti twice daily. This stovetop recipe made in a stockpot is an easy version of the casserole that bears her name.

Ingredients

10 to 12 oz frozen chopped broccoli
2 TBSP olive oil or vegetable oil
2 TBSP butter
1 lb boneless skinless chicken breast or thigh meat, cut into 1/2" cubes
8 oz white button mushrooms, sliced
2 TBSP dried onion flakes
1 tsp salt
1/4 tsp black pepper
1 tsp thyme, dried
1/2 tsp ground sage
1 TBSP dried parsley flakes
1 tsp granulated garlic *
1/2 cup white wine (substitute water)
2 1/2 cups gluten-free chicken broth *
12 oz corn and rice blend gluten-free spaghetti **
3/4 cup grated Parmesan cheese *
1 cup half-and-half

* See *Tips* section
** Use a gluten-free spaghetti that is made from a corn and rice blend instead of 100% rice. The corn will keep the spaghetti from becoming gummy as it cooks.

Cookware and Utensils

6-quart stockpot with lid
Colander
Small bowl
Shredder/grater
   (if not using pre-grated cheese)

Instructions

1. Transfer the frozen broccoli to the countertop to thaw.

2. Add the oil and the butter to the stockpot. Heat on low heat to melt the butter. While the butter is melting cut the chicken into 1/2-inch cubes. Add the chicken to the stockpot. Stir to coat the chicken with the butter and the oil. Cover the stockpot with the lid. Increase the heat to medium low and cook, covered, until the chicken is fully cooked (opaque all the way through when cut with a knife). Stir occasionally.

3. Rinse the mushrooms in the colander. Drain thoroughly. Slice the mushrooms. When the chicken is fully cooked add the mushrooms to the stockpot. Stir to combine. Cover the stockpot with the lid. Increase the heat to medium and cook, covered, until the mushrooms are soft. Stir occasionally.

4. Add the dried onion flakes, salt, pepper, thyme, sage, dried parsley flakes, and garlic to the small bowl. Stir to combine. When the mushrooms are soft add the mixed seasonings to the stockpot. Stir to coat the chicken and mushrooms with the seasonings. Add the white wine (substitute water) and the chicken broth to the stockpot. Stir to combine.

5. Break the gluten-free spaghetti in half. Add the spaghetti to the stockpot in a crisscross pattern, a few strands at a time, distributing it evenly to keep the spaghetti strands from sticking to each other. Use a large-bowl spoon to scoop the liquid over the spaghetti to moisten and submerge the spaghetti in the liquid. Cover the stockpot with the lid. Increase the heat to medium high until the liquid begins to boil then reduce the heat to a gentle simmer. After the spaghetti begins to soften use a fork to gently separate any strands that have stuck together. Cover the stockpot with the lid. Simmer, stirring occasionally, until the spaghetti is 'al dente' (soft but with 'a bite'). While the spaghetti is cooking grate the Parmesan cheese (if not using pre-grated cheese).

6. When the spaghetti is done add the half-and-half and the broccoli to the stockpot. Stir to combine. Sprinkle the cheese over the stockpot. Stir to combine. Cook, covered, on medium low heat to melt the cheese. Stir gently to combine. Serve immediately.

Chipotle Chicken and Rice

This recipe is a variation on Arroz Con Pollo (Chicken with Rice), a traditional Latino recipe. Smoked chipotle chili, tangy lime, and lots of garlic turns a normally bland dish into a meal that's bursting with flavor. Serve this dish with (optional) warm corn tortillas and sliced avocado so diners can make their own chicken tacos if desired.

Ingredients

2 TBSP vegetable oil
6 bone-in, skin-on chicken thighs
1 large onion, sliced into crescents
4 cloves garlic, chopped
2 TBSP lime juice (about 2 limes)
3/4 tsp salt
1 tsp oregano, dried (use Mexican oregano for extra flavor)
1/2 tsp cayenne pepper
1 1/2 tsp ground cumin
1 1/2 tsp ground chipotle chili
1 15-oz can tomatoes, diced or crushed (do not drain)
1 1/2 cups long grain white rice
2 1/2 cups water

For the optional tacos

12 corn tortillas
1 avocado, peeled, pit removed, sliced

Instructions

1. If serving the (optional) warm tortillas then preheat the oven to 200 degrees F. Stack corn tortillas on the bottom of an oven-proof casserole dish, staggering them slightly so they do not stick to each other. Cover the casserole dish with its lid or aluminum foil. Transfer the casserole dish to the oven to warm the tortillas while you prepare the chicken and rice.

2. Add the oil to the skillet. Heat the oil on medium heat until it begins to bubble.

3. While the oil is heating rinse the chicken thighs and pat them dry with clean paper towels. When the oil is hot use the kitchen tongs to transfer the chicken thighs to the skillet. Brown the chicken thighs on medium heat, turning once to brown both sides. Brown the chicken until it is cooked at least halfway through.

4. While the chicken is browning chop the onion and the garlic.

5. Juice the limes.

6. When the chicken thighs are browned and cooked halfway through transfer them to a clean dinner plate. Add the onion and garlic to the skillet. Stir to coat the onion and the garlic with the pan drippings. Cover the skillet with the lid. Continue cooking on medium heat, stirring occasionally, until the onion is soft.

7. When the onion is soft add the salt, oregano, cayenne pepper, cumin, and chipotle chili to the skillet. Stir to coat the vegetables with the seasonings.

8. Add the tomatoes (do not drain) to the skillet. Stir to combine.

9. Add the rice to the skillet. Stir to coat the rice with the tomatoes and seasonings.

10. Add the water and the lime juice to the skillet. Stir to combine.

Continued

Chipotle Chicken and Rice
- Continued -

Cookware and Utensils

Oven-proof casserole dish (optional)
12-inch skillet with lid
Kitchen tongs
Citrus juicer
Dinner plate

Instructions - continued

11. Transfer the browned chicken thighs to the skillet, layering them evenly over the rice mixture. Cover the skillet with the lid. Increase the heat to medium high until the liquid boils then reduce the heat to a gentle simmer.

12. Simmer the chicken and rice, covered, until the rice is tender and the water is fully absorbed. Test the chicken for doneness. Fully cooked chicken will be opaque in the middle when cut with a knife. If the chicken is not fully cooked reduce the heat to low and continue cooking, covered, until the chicken is cooked all the way through.

13. If serving the (optional) sliced avocado then peel, pit, and slice the avocado. At serving time transfer the skillet, sliced avocado, and warm tortillas to the dinner table. Let diners help themselves by scooping seasoned rice onto a warm tortilla, adding some shredded chicken, topping with a slice of avocado, and rolling into a taco.

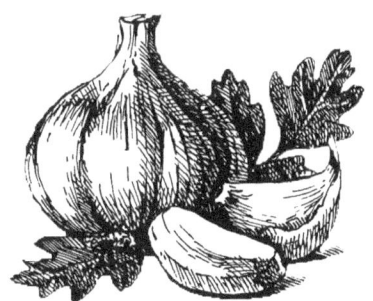

Classic Chicken Noodle Soup

Nothing says 'comfort food' like a steaming bowl of Chicken Noodle Soup. This version of the classic comfort food is loaded with lots of meaty chicken and vegetables. Making a gluten-free Chicken Noodle Soup can be a challenge because gluten is the sticky substance that holds the noodles together and keeps them from falling apart in the hot broth. The trick to making a gluten-free Chicken Noodle Soup is to add the noodles when the soup is almost done.

Ingredients

1 quart gluten-free chicken broth *
3 cups water
1 lb skinless boneless chicken breast or thigh meat, cut into 1/2" cubes
1 cup onion, chopped (about 1/2 of a large onion)
1 TBSP vegetable oil
2 tsp salt
1/4 tsp black pepper
1/2 tsp marjoram, dried
2 tsp dried parsley flakes
1 bay leaf
4 carrots, ends trimmed and cut into 1/2" rounds
4 ribs celery, ends trimmed and sliced into 1/2" pieces
7 to 8 oz Pad Thai-style rice noodles, broken in half

* See *Tips* section

Cookware and Utensils

6-quart stockpot with lid

Instructions

1. Add the chicken broth and 3 cups of water to the stockpot. Heat on medium high heat.

2. While the broth is heating cut the chicken into 1/2-inch cubes. Add the chicken to the stockpot. Stir to combine.

3. Chop the onion. Add the onion to the stockpot. Stir to combine.

4. Add the vegetable oil to the stockpot. Stir to combine.

5. Add the salt, pepper, marjoram, parsley, and the bay leaf to the stockpot. Stir to combine.

6. Scrub the carrots under running water, trim their ends, and slice them into 1/2-inch rounds. Add the carrots to the stockpot. Stir to combine.

7. Rinse the celery ribs and trim their ends. Slice each rib into 1/2-inch thick slices. Add the celery to the stockpot. Stir to combine. Cover the stockpot with the lid. Heat on medium high heat until the broth boils then reduce the heat to a gentle simmer. Simmer the soup, covered, until the carrots pierce easily with the tines of a fork.

8. When the carrots are tender remove the bay leaf. Break the Pad Thai noodles in half and add them to the stockpot. Submerge the noodles below the broth. Wait a few minutes for the noodles to soften then stir them with a fork to separate them. Cover the stockpot with the lid and shut off the heat. Allow the noodles to cook in the hot broth until they are soft.

9. When the noodles are soft the soup is done. Serve the soup hot.

White Bean Chili with Chicken and Red Onion

This easy white bean chili is made with chicken and is ideal for those who prefer chicken instead of beef. Tangy red onion and jalapeno peppers give it flavor. Canned chilies, canned white beans, and convenient jar salsa make this recipe quick and easy. This recipe uses salsa verde (green salsa) which is a mild salsa made from green tomatillos.

Ingredients

1 lb boneless skinless chicken breast or thigh meat, cut into 3/4" cubes
2 TBSP vegetable oil
1 1/2 cups red onion, sliced into crescents
1 bell pepper (red, green, or yellow), seeded and diced into 1/2" pieces
1 4-oz can diced mild green chilis (do not drain)
1 4-oz can diced jalapeno peppers (do not drain), use 2 TBSP peppers, add additional to taste
1/2 tsp salt
1 tsp oregano, dried
1 1/2 tsp ground cumin
1/4 tsp ground sage
1 24-oz jar salsa verde (green salsa made with tomatillos)
3 15-oz cans white beans (Cannellini, Great Northern, Navy, or other white beans), rinsed and drained
1 cup cilantro leaves (about 1 medium bunch)

Optional Garnish

1 cup shredded Monterey Jack cheese *
  (about 4 oz by weight)

* See *Tips* section

Cookware and Utensils

6-quart stockpot with lid
Colander
Shredder/grater
  (if not using pre-shredded cheese)

Instructions

1. Cut the chicken into 3/4-inch cubes. Add the chicken and the oil to the stockpot. Stir to coat the chicken with the oil. Cook on medium heat, stirring occasionally.

2. Slice the onion into crescents. Seed and dice the bell pepper into 1/2-inch pieces. When the chicken is fully cooked (opaque all the way through when cut with a knife) add the onion and bell pepper to the stockpot. Stir to combine. Cook, stirring occasionally, until the onion is soft.

3. When the onion is soft add the mild green chilis to the stockpot (do not drain). Stir to combine. Measure 2 tablespoons of the diced jalapeno peppers and add them to the stockpot. Stir to combine. Reserve the unused portion to adjust the level of heat after all ingredients have been added.

4. Add the salt, oregano, cumin, and sage to the stockpot. Stir to combine. Add the salsa verde to the stockpot. Stir to combine. Rinse the beans in the colander and allow them to drain. Add the beans to the stockpot. Stir to combine.

5. Taste the chili for seasoning balance. If a hotter chili is desired add more diced jalapeno peppers to the chili, mixing in increments of 1 tablespoon until the chili is hot enough for your taste. Transfer the unused portion of jalapeno peppers to a non-metal container and store in the freezer. Jalapeno peppers may be stored in the freezer for up to one month.

6. After you have adjusted the heat level of the chili cover the stockpot with the lid. Increase the heat to medium high until the chili boils then reduce the heat to a gentle simmer. Stir occasionally.

7. Rinse and drain the cilantro in the colander. Remove the leaves from the stems until you have enough cilantro leaves to yield 1 cup. Coarsely chop the cilantro leaves and add them to the stockpot. Stir to combine. Cover the stockpot with the lid and continue simmering the chili for 10 minutes to combine flavors. While the chili is simmering shred the (optional) Monterey Jack cheese.

8. Serve the chili hot. Top the chili with (optional) shredded Monterey Jack cheese if desired.

California Rancho Posole

California ranchos were large tracts of land settled by Mexican and Spanish cowboys who cooked their meals over an open fire at the end of the day. Posole is a traditional rancho soup made with slow-simmered chicken or pork, chili seasonings, and hominy (corn kernels processed with lime to remove their hulls). This recipe uses flavorful chipotle chili powder that lends a smoky wood fire taste to a traditional cowboy meal.

Ingredients

1 lb boneless skinless chicken breast or thigh meat, cut into 3/4" cubes (substitute boneless pork shoulder)
1 TBSP vegetable oil
1 cup onion, chopped (about 1/2 of a large onion)
1/2 tsp salt
1/4 tsp black pepper
1/2 tsp oregano, dried (use Mexican oregano for extra flavor)
1/2 tsp ground cumin
1 tsp granulated garlic *
1 tsp chili powder *
1 tsp ground chipotle chili
1 quart gluten-free chicken broth *
1 25-oz or 30-oz can hominy, rinsed and drained
1 bay leaf
1 15-oz can tomatoes, diced or crushed (do not drain)

* See *Tips* section

Cookware and Utensils

6-quart stockpot with lid
Small bowl
Colander

Instructions

1. Cut the chicken (or pork) into 3/4-inch cubes.

2. Add the chicken (or pork) and the oil to the stockpot. Stir to combine. Cook on medium heat, stirring occasionally, until the meat is fully cooked. When fully cooked the chicken will be opaque all the way through when cut with a knife. When fully cooked the pork will not have any pink color when cut with a knife.

3. While the meat is cooking chop the onion.

4. After the meat has fully cooked add the onion to the stockpot. Stir to combine. Continue cooking on medium heat, stirring occasionally, until the onion is soft.

5. Add the salt, pepper, oregano, cumin, garlic, chili powder, and chipotle chili to the small bowl. Stir to combine. Add the mixed seasonings to the meat and onion mixture. Stir to coat the meat and onions with the seasonings.

6. Add the chicken broth to the stockpot. Stir to combine.

7. Rinse the hominy in the colander and allow it to drain thoroughly. Add the hominy to the stockpot. Stir to combine.

8. Add the bay leaf and the tomatoes (do not drain) to the stockpot. Stir to combine. Cover the stockpot with the lid. Increase the heat to medium high until the soup boils then decrease the heat to a gentle simmer.

9. Simmer the soup, covered, for 20 minutes to combine flavors. Stir occasionally.

10. After the soup has simmered for 20 minutes remove the bay leaf. Serve the soup hot.

Chicken and Rice Soup

This easy chicken soup is a bowlful of comfort food that is perfect for a rainy weekend when you're not feeling well or a Snow Day when school gets let out unexpectedly. It uses pre-packaged chicken broth for convenience and converted (parboiled) rice which keeps its shape and won't become mushy as the soup cooks.

Ingredients

1 quart gluten-free chicken broth *
1 1/2 cups water
1 1/2 tsp salt
1/4 tsp black pepper
1 TBSP dried parsley flakes
1/2 tsp marjoram, dried
1/2 tsp thyme, dried
1 tsp granulated garlic *
1 bay leaf
1 lb skinless boneless chicken breast
   or thigh meat, cut into 1/2" cubes
1 cup onion, chopped
   (about 1/2 of a large onion)
3 carrots, scrubbed, ends trimmed,
   halved lengthwise, each half sliced
   into 3/8" thick slices
3 ribs celery, ends trimmed,
   halved lengthwise, each half sliced
   into 3/8" thick slices
1/2 cup converted (parboiled) rice **
1 TBSP vegetable oil

* See **Tips** section
** See **Converted Rice** section

Cookware and Utensils

6-quart stockpot with lid
Small bowl

Instructions

1. Add the chicken broth and the water to the stockpot. Heat on medium high heat until the broth boils then reduce the heat to a gentle simmer.

2. While the broth is heating add the salt, pepper, parsley, marjoram, thyme, garlic, and the bay leaf to the stockpot. Stir to combine.

3. Cut the chicken into 1/2-inch cubes. Add the chicken to the stockpot. Stir to combine. Cover the stockpot with the lid and continue to simmer the soup as you prepare the vegetables.

4. Chop the onion. Add the onion to the stockpot. Stir to combine.

5. Scrub the carrots under running water and trim their ends. Slice each carrot in half lengthwise. Slice each half into 3/8-inch thick slices. Add the carrots to the stockpot. Stir to combine.

6. Wash and trim the ends of the celery. Slice each rib of celery in half lengthwise. Slice the halved celery ribs into 3/8-inch thick slices. Add the celery to the stockpot. Stir to combine.

7. Add the converted (parboiled) rice to the small bowl.

8. Pour the oil over the rice. Stir to coat the rice with the oil. Add the oil-coated rice to the stockpot. Stir the soup to evenly disperse the rice.

9. Cover the stockpot with the lid. Increase the heat to medium high until the soup boils then reduce the heat to a gentle simmer. Stir occasionally. Simmer until the rice is fully cooked and the carrots pierce easily with the tines of a fork.

10. When the rice and carrots are fully cooked remove the bay leaf. Serve the soup hot.

Southwestern Chicken Stew

This hearty chicken stew takes its cues from the flavors of the American Southwest. Green chili, cilantro, lime, red onion, and bell pepper add flavor while red pepper flakes and cayenne pepper add just enough heat. Try this stew with our gluten-free cornbread muffin recipe.

Ingredients

1 1/2 lbs boneless skinless chicken breast
   or thigh meat, cut into 3/4" cubes
2 TBSP vegetable oil
2 cups red onion, sliced into crescents
1 red bell pepper, diced into 1/2" pieces
1 tsp salt
1 tsp oregano, dried
   (use Mexican oregano if available)
1 1/2 tsp ground cumin
1/2 tsp ground coriander
1/4 tsp ground sage
1/4 tsp cayenne pepper
1/2 tsp hot red pepper flakes
2 tsp granulated garlic *
1 4-oz can diced mild green chilis
   (do not drain)
3 cups gluten-free chicken broth *
   (reserve 1 cup)
3 TBSP cornstarch
4 carrots, ends trimmed,
   sliced into 1/2" thick slices
1 1/2 lbs potatoes, cut into 1" cubes
2 limes juiced (about 2 TBSP juice)
1 cup cilantro leaves, coarsely chopped
   (about 1 medium bunch)

* See *Tips* section

Instructions

1. Cut the chicken into 3/4-inch cubes.

2. Add the chicken and the oil to the stockpot. Stir to combine. Heat on medium heat, stirring frequently, until the chicken is fully cooked (opaque all the way through when cut with a knife).

3. While the chicken is cooking slice the onion into crescents.

4. Wash and seed the bell pepper. Dice the bell pepper into 1/2-inch pieces.

5. Add the salt, oregano, cumin, coriander, sage, cayenne pepper, red pepper flakes, and the garlic to the small bowl. Stir to combine.

6. When the chicken is fully cooked add the onion and the bell pepper to the stockpot. Stir to combine. Continue cooking on medium heat, stirring occasionally, until the onion is soft.

7. When the onion is soft add the diced mild green chilis to the stockpot (do not drain). Stir to combine.

8. Add the mixed seasonings to the stockpot. Stir to coat the chicken and vegetable mixture with the seasonings.

9. Add 2 cups of the chicken broth to the stockpot. Stir to combine.

10. Pour the reserved cup of chicken broth into the liquid measuring cup. Add the cornstarch to the chicken broth. Stir with a fork to completely dissolve the cornstarch. Slowly pour the broth and cornstarch mixture into the stockpot. Stir to combine.

11. Scrub the carrots under running water, trim their ends, and slice them into 1/2-inch thick slices. Add the carrots to the stockpot. Stir to combine.

Continued

Southwestern Chicken Stew
- Continued -

Cookware and Utensils

6-quart stockpot with lid
Small bowl
2-cup liquid measuring cup
Citrus juicer
Colander

Instructions - continued

12. Scrub the potatoes under running water. Cut the potatoes into 1-inch cubes. Add the potatoes to the stockpot. Stir to combine. Cover the stockpot with the lid. Increase the heat to medium high until the stew boils then reduce the heat to a gentle simmer. Simmer the stew, covered, until the carrots and potatoes pierce easily with the tines of a fork.

13. While the stew is simmering juice the limes. Add the lime juice to the stockpot. Stir to combine.

14. Rinse the cilantro in the colander. Remove the stems from the cilantro until you have enough cilantro leaves to yield 1 cup. Coarsely chop the cilantro leaves. Add the cilantro leaves to the stockpot. Stir to combine. Continue simmering until the vegetables are tender.

15. When the potatoes and carrots pierce easily with the tines of a fork the stew is done. Serve the stew hot.

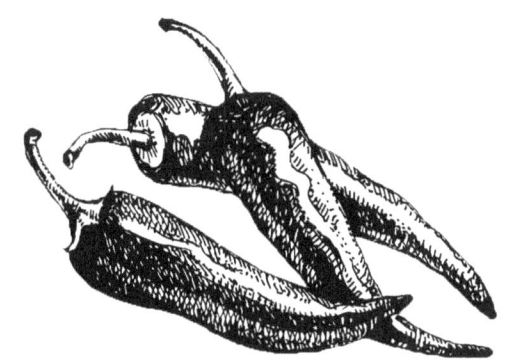

Chicken and Vegetable Bean Soup

This quick and easy soup is ready in no time and is light on the calories while providing a full serving of vegetables in every bowl. Lean chicken and lots of herbs give it flavor while packaged chicken broth, canned beans, and frozen mixed vegetables provide convenience.

Ingredients

10 to 12 oz frozen mixed vegetables
1 quart gluten-free chicken broth *
1 TBSP vegetable oil
1 1/2 tsp salt
1/4 tsp black pepper
1 TBSP dried parsley flakes
1/2 tsp marjoram, dried
1/4 tsp thyme, dried
1/4 tsp oregano, dried
1 tsp granulated garlic *
1 bay leaf
1 lb boneless skinless chicken breast or thigh meat, cut into 1/2" cubes
1 1/2 cups onion, chopped
1 15-oz can white beans (Cannellini, Great Northern, Navy, or other white beans), rinsed and drained

* See *Tips* section

Cookware and Utensils

6-quart stockpot with lid
Colander

Instructions

1. Transfer the frozen mixed vegetables to the countertop to thaw while you are making the soup.

2. Add the chicken broth, oil, salt, pepper, parsley, marjoram, thyme, oregano, garlic, and the bay leaf to the stockpot. Stir to combine. Cover the stockpot with the lid. Heat on medium high heat until the broth boils then reduce the heat to a gentle simmer.

3. Cut the chicken into 1/2-inch cubes. Add the chicken to the stockpot. Stir to combine.

4. Chop the onion. Add the onion to the stockpot. Stir to combine.

5. Rinse the beans in the colander and allow them to drain thoroughly. Add the beans to the stockpot. Stir to combine.

6. Add the frozen vegetables to the stockpot. Stir to combine. Cover the stockpot with the lid. Increase the heat to medium high until the soup boils then reduce the heat to a gentle simmer. Simmer, covered, for 15 minutes to combine flavors. Stir occasionally.

7. After the soup has simmered for 15 minutes remove the bay leaf. Serve the soup hot.

Santa Fe Soup

This hearty soup features the colors and flavors of the Southwest - red bell pepper and tomato, yellow corn, green chili peppers, and black beans. Meaty chicken, green chilis, and bell pepper add flavor. A medley of rice, black beans, and corn makes it a filling one-pot meal. Pair this soup with our gluten-free cornbread muffin recipe for an authentic Southwest meal.

Ingredients

1 lb boneless skinless chicken breast or thigh meat, cut into 1/2" cubes
2 TBSP vegetable oil
1 1/2 cups red onion, sliced into crescents
1 red bell pepper, seeded and diced into 1/2" pieces
3 carrots, ends trimmed, sliced into 3/8" thick rounds
1 4-oz can diced mild green chilis (do not drain)
1 3/4 tsp salt
2 tsp ground cumin
1 tsp oregano, dried
1/2 tsp rosemary, dried
1/2 tsp thyme, dried
1/2 tsp marjoram, dried
1 TBSP chili powder *
1 1/2 tsp granulated garlic *
1/4 tsp hot red pepper flakes
1 quart gluten-free chicken broth *
1/2 cup converted (parboiled) rice **
1 15-oz can black beans, rinsed and drained
1 15-oz can tomatoes, crushed or diced (do not drain)
1 cup frozen corn kernels

* See *Tips* section
** See *Converted Rice* section

Cookware and Utensils

6-quart stockpot with lid
Colander

Instructions

1. Cut the chicken into 1/2-inch cubes.

2. Add the chicken and the oil to the stockpot. Stir to combine. Cook on medium heat, stirring occasionally, until the chicken is fully cooked (opaque all the way through when cut with a knife).

3. While the chicken is cooking slice the red onion into crescents.

4. Wash and seed the bell pepper. Dice the bell pepper into 1/2-inch pieces.

5. Scrub the carrots under running water, trim their ends, and slice them into 3/8-inch thick rounds.

6. When the chicken is fully cooked add the red onion, bell pepper, and carrots to the stockpot. Stir to combine. Continue cooking on medium heat, stirring occasionally, until the red onion is soft.

7. When the red onion is soft add the green chilis to the stockpot (do not drain). Stir to combine.

8. Add the salt, cumin, oregano, rosemary, thyme, marjoram, chili powder, garlic, and the red pepper flakes to the stockpot. Stir to coat the chicken and vegetables with the seasonings.

9. Add the chicken broth and the converted (parboiled) rice to the stockpot. Stir to combine.

10. Rinse the black beans in the colander and allow them to drain thoroughly. Add the black beans to the stockpot. Stir gently to combine.

11. Add the tomatoes (do not drain) and the corn kernels to the stockpot. Stir to combine. Cover the stockpot with the lid. Increase the heat to medium high until the soup boils then reduce the heat to a gentle simmer. Stir occasionally.

12. Simmer the soup, covered, until the carrots pierce easily with the tines of a fork and the rice is fully cooked. Serve the soup hot.

Chicken and Summer Vegetable Stew

In early summer zucchini and summer squash are abundant. This savory chicken and summer vegetable stew takes advantage of this abundance and is perfect for a light supper. Herbs, garlic, and white wine add flavor while meaty mushrooms and lots of chicken make it a satisfying meal.

Ingredients

1 1/2 lbs boneless skinless chicken breast or thigh meat, cut into 1" cubes
2 TBSP vegetable oil
2 cups onion, sliced into crescents
3 cloves garlic, chopped
8 oz white button mushrooms, sliced
3/4 tsp salt
1/4 tsp pepper
1/2 tsp thyme, dried
1/2 tsp oregano, dried
1/2 tsp basil, dried (substitute 1 TBSP fresh basil cut into ribbons)
1 tsp dried parsley flakes (substitute 2 TBSP fresh parsley, coarsely chopped)
1/2 cup white wine (substitute water)
2 cups gluten-free chicken broth *
3 TBSP cornstarch
3 carrots, ends trimmed, sliced into 1/2" thick rounds
1 zucchini, sliced in half lengthwise, halves sliced into 1/2" thick slices
1 yellow summer squash, sliced in half lengthwise, halves sliced into 1/2" thick slices

* See *Tips* section

Instructions

1. Cut the chicken into 1-inch cubes.

2. Add the chicken and the oil to the stockpot. Stir to combine. Cover the stockpot with the lid. Cook on medium heat, stirring occasionally, until the chicken is fully cooked (opaque all the way through when cut with a knife).

3. While the chicken is cooking slice the onion into crescents.

4. Chop the garlic.

5. Rinse the mushrooms in the colander and allow them to drain thoroughly. Slice the mushrooms.

6. When the chicken is fully cooked add the onion, garlic, and mushrooms to the stockpot. Stir to combine. Cover the stockpot with the lid. Cook on medium heat, stirring occasionally, until the onion and mushrooms are soft.

7. When the onion and mushrooms are soft add the salt, pepper, thyme, oregano, basil, and the parsley to the stockpot. Stir to coat the chicken and the vegetables with the seasonings.

8. Add the white wine (substitute water) to the stockpot. Stir to combine.

9. Measure the chicken broth into the liquid measuring cup or bowl. Add the cornstarch to the chicken broth. Stir with a fork to completely dissolve the cornstarch into the broth. Slowly add the broth to the stockpot, stirring the stew continuously to avoid clumping the cornstarch.

10. Scrub the carrots under running water, trim their ends, and slice them into 1/2-inch thick rounds. Add the carrots to the stockpot. Stir to combine.

Continued

Chicken and Summer Vegetable Stew
- Continued -

Cookware and Utensils

6-quart stockpot with lid
Colander
2-cup liquid measuring cup
 (or larger) or medium bowl

Instructions - continued

11. Wash the zucchini and summer squash and trim their ends. Slice the zucchini and summer squash in half lengthwise. Slice the halves of the zucchini and the summer squash into 1/2-inch thick slices. Add the zucchini and the summer squash to the stockpot. Stir to combine. Cover the stockpot with the lid. Increase the heat to medium high until the stew boils then reduce the heat to a gentle simmer.

12. Simmer the stew, covered, until the carrots pierce easily with the tines of a fork. Stir occasionally.

13. When the vegetables are tender crisp the stew is done. Do not overcook or the zucchini and the summer squash will become mushy. Serve immediately.

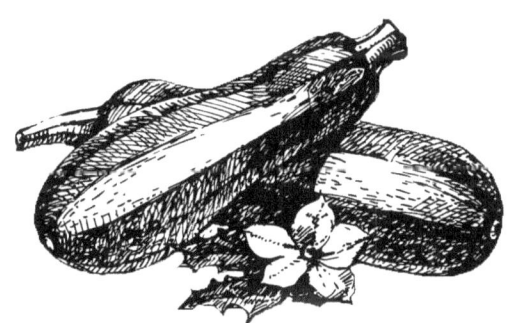

Moroccan Chicken and Apricot Stew

A tagine (pronounced 'tah-JHEEN' like the French word for eggplant 'aubergine') is a traditional Moroccan stew cooked over a charcoal fire in a ceramic pot that has a cone-shaped lid. The conical shape of the lid allows steam to condense and drip back down into the pot keeping the meat and vegetables moist during cooking.

Ingredients

1 1/2 lbs boneless skinless chicken breast or thigh meat, cut into 3/4" cubes
2 TBSP vegetable oil
2 cups onion, chopped (about 1 large onion)
1 lb carrots, trimmed and cut into 1" lengths
1 lb sweet potatoes or yams, peeled and cut into 1" cubes
1/2 tsp salt
1/4 tsp black pepper
1 1/2 tsp ground coriander
1 1/2 tsp ground cumin
1 tsp turmeric
1/2 tsp paprika
1 1/2 tsp granulated garlic *
1/4 tsp cinnamon
1 TBSP + 1 tsp honey
2 cups gluten-free chicken broth *
1 TBSP fresh ginger, grated (substitute 1 TBSP ginger paste or 1/2 tsp ground ginger)
6 oz dried apricots, cut into quarters (about 1 cup chopped)
1 15-oz can tomatoes, diced or crushed (do not drain)
1 15-oz can chickpeas (garbanzo beans), rinsed and drained
1 TBSP Harissa paste (optional – omit this if you don't like your stew spicy)
* See *Tips* section

Optional Garnishes
Cilantro leaves
Flat Leaf Parsley

Instructions

1. Dice the chicken into 3/4-inch cubes.

2. Add the chicken and the oil to the stockpot. Stir to coat the chicken with the oil. Cook on medium heat until the chicken is fully cooked (opaque all the way through when cut with a knife). Stir occasionally.

3. While the chicken is cooking chop the onion. Add the onion to the stockpot. Stir to combine.

4. Scrub the carrots under running water and trim their ends. Cut the carrots into 1-inch lengths.

5. Peel the sweet potato (or yam). Cut the sweet potato (or yam) into 1-inch cubes.

6. When the chicken is fully cooked add the carrots and the sweet potato (or yam) to the stockpot. Stir to combine. Continue cooking on medium heat, stirring occasionally.

7. Add the salt, pepper, coriander, cumin, turmeric, paprika, garlic, and cinnamon to the small bowl. Stir to combine. Add the mixed seasonings to the stockpot. Stir to combine.

8. Add the honey to the stockpot. Stir to combine.

9. Add the chicken broth to the stockpot. Stir to combine.

10. Peel about 2 inches of fresh ginger root. Use the fine holes of a shredder/grater to grate 1 tablespoon of fresh ginger root. Add the grated ginger root to the stockpot. Stir to combine. You may substitute 1 tablespoon of ginger paste or 1/2 teaspoon of ground ginger instead of fresh ginger.

11. Cut the dried apricots into quarters. Add the apricots to the stockpot. Stir to combine.

12. Add the tomatoes to the stockpot (do not drain). Stir to combine.

13. Drain and rinse the chickpeas (garbanzo beans) in a colander. Allow the chickpeas to drain thoroughly then add them to the stockpot. Stir to combine.

Continued

Moroccan Chicken and Apricot Stew
- Continued -

This chicken and apricot stew recipe is based on traditional Moroccan tagine recipes. If you like your stew mild then skip the addition of the Harissa paste which can be found in the international foods section at your grocer.

Cookware and Utensils

6-quart stockpot with lid
Vegetable peeler or paring knife
Small bowl
Shredder/grater (if using fresh ginger)
Colander

Instructions - continued

14. Taste the stew for flavoring. If you like your stew sweet and savory then omit the Harissa paste. If you like a spicy stew then add the Harissa paste to the stockpot. Stir to combine.

15. Cover the stockpot with the lid. Increase the heat to medium high until the stew boils then reduce the heat to a gentle simmer. Simmer the stew for 20 minutes to combine flavors. Stir occasionally.

16. After 20 minutes of simmering pierce a carrot and sweet potato with the tines of a fork. If the vegetables do not pierce easily continue simmering, covered, for an additional 10 minutes or until the vegetables are tender.

17. Serve the stew hot with honey and (optional) Harissa paste on the side so diners may mix the honey and Harissa paste into the stew to their desired sweetness and heat level. Traditional garnishes are cilantro leaves or flat leaf parsley.

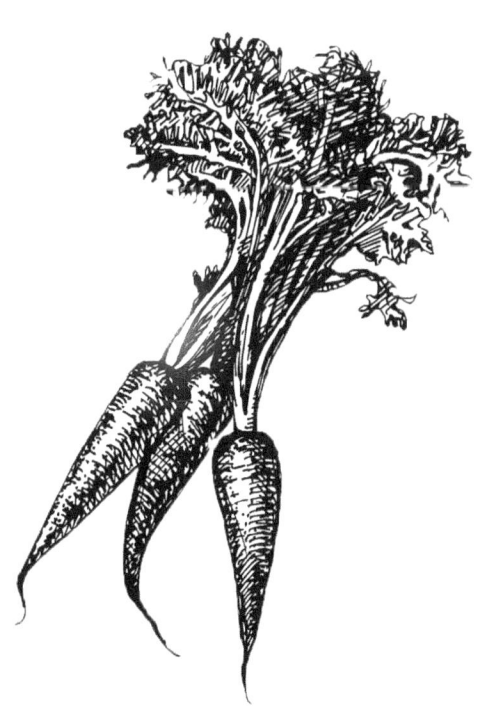

Italian Hunter's Chicken

In Italian the word 'cacciatore' means 'hunter'. Chicken Cacciatore or 'Hunter's Chicken' has its origins in the simple dishes prepared from foods that hunters could gather in the woods. Originally made with rabbit and foraged mushrooms and herbs, the modern incarnation of this dish substitutes easier-to-find chicken and adds tomatoes and vegetables foraged from your grocer's produce department.

Ingredients

2 TBSP vegetable oil
8 skin-on, bone-in chicken thighs
  and/or drumsticks
1 cup onion, chopped
  (about 1/2 of a large onion)
4 garlic cloves, chopped
1 green bell pepper,
  seeded and diced into 1/2" pieces
2 carrots, ends trimmed,
  cut in half lengthwise,
  each half sliced into 3/8" thick slices
2 ribs celery, ends trimmed,
  sliced into 3/8" thick slices
8 oz white button mushrooms, sliced
1 tsp salt
1/4 tsp black pepper
3/4 tsp oregano, dried
1/2 tsp basil, dried
1/2 tsp hot red pepper flakes
1 28-oz can tomatoes, diced or crushed
  (do not drain)
1/2 cup white wine (substitute water)

Instructions

1. Add the oil to the stockpot. Heat the oil on medium heat until it begins to bubble.

2. While the oil is heating rinse the chicken and pat it dry with clean paper towels.

3. When the oil is hot use the kitchen tongs to transfer half of the chicken to the stockpot. Brown the chicken on medium heat, turning once to brown both sides.

4. While the chicken is browning chop the onion and the garlic.

5. Wash and seed the bell pepper. Dice the bell pepper into 1/2-inch pieces.

6. When the first half of the chicken is browned transfer it to a clean dinner plate and repeat the browning process with the remaining uncooked chicken.

7. While the chicken is browning scrub the carrots under running water, trim their ends, and slice each carrot in half lengthwise. Slice each half into 3/8-inch thick slices.

8. Wash the celery ribs, trim their ends, and slice each rib into 3/8-inch thick slices.

9. Rinse the mushrooms in the colander and allow them to drain thoroughly. Slice the mushrooms.

10. When the rest of the chicken has browned transfer it to the dinner plate. Add the onion, garlic, bell pepper, carrots, celery, and mushrooms to the stockpot. Stir to coat the vegetables with the pan drippings. Cover the stockpot with the lid. Cook on medium heat, stirring occasionally, until the onion and mushrooms are soft.

11. When the onion and mushrooms are soft add the salt, pepper, oregano, basil, and hot pepper flakes to the stockpot. Stir to coat the vegetables with the seasonings.

Continued

Italian Hunter's Chicken
Cover Photo Recipe
- Continued -

Cookware and Utensils

6-quart stockpot with lid
Kitchen tongs
Dinner plate
Colander
4 wide and shallow serving bowls

Instructions - continued

12. Add the tomatoes (do not drain) and the white wine (substitute water) to the stockpot. Stir to combine.

13. Use the kitchen tongs to transfer the browned chicken to the stockpot, layering it evenly in the stockpot. Spoon the tomato and vegetable mixture over the chicken. Cover the stockpot with the lid. Increase the heat to medium high until the liquid boils then reduce the heat to a gentle simmer.

14. Simmer the chicken, covered, until it is fully cooked (about 30 minutes). Fully cooked chicken will be opaque in the middle when cut with a knife. Serve the stew hot in bowls. Use the tongs to transfer the chicken to the bowls then spoon the sauce over the chicken. Serve immediately.

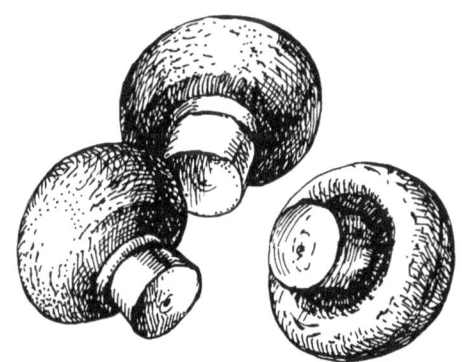

Chunky Cream of Chicken and Mushroom Soup

This easy soup is loaded with chicken and mushrooms and gets extra flavor from herbs and just a hint of garlic. For a more intense and earthy mushroom flavor substitute cremini (baby portobello) mushrooms instead of the more common white button mushrooms.

Ingredients

4 TBSP butter
1 lb boneless skinless chicken breast or thigh meat, cut into 1/2" cubes
1/3 cup onion, finely diced
16 oz white button mushrooms, washed and sliced/diced (substitute cremini mushrooms)
1 tsp salt
1/4 tsp black pepper
1/2 tsp thyme, dried
3/4 tsp granulated garlic *
2 cups gluten-free chicken broth *
2/3 cup mashed potato flakes
2 cups half-and-half

* See *Tips* section

Cookware and Utensils

6-quart stockpot with lid
Colander

Instructions

1. Add the butter to the stockpot. Melt the butter on low heat.

2. While the butter is melting cut the chicken into 1/2-inch cubes. Add the chicken to the stockpot. Stir to combine. Cover the stockpot with the lid. Increase the heat to medium low and continue cooking, stirring occasionally, until the chicken is fully cooked (opaque all the way through when cut with a knife).

3. Finely dice the onion. When the chicken is fully cooked add the onion to the stockpot. Stir to combine.

4. Rinse and drain the mushrooms in the colander. Dice half of the mushrooms into 3/8-inch cubes. Slice the other half of the mushrooms. Add the mushrooms to the stockpot. Stir to coat the mushrooms with the chicken, onions, and butter. Cover the stockpot with the lid. Increase the heat to medium and cook, stirring occasionally, until the mushrooms are soft.

5. When the mushrooms are soft add the salt, pepper, thyme, and garlic to the stockpot. Stir to combine.

6. Add the chicken broth to the stockpot. Stir to combine. Increase the heat to medium high until the broth boils then reduce the heat to a gentle simmer.

7. When the broth is gently simmering sprinkle the mashed potato flakes over the soup. Stir to combine. Allow the flakes to rehydrate for a minute or two then stir the soup again to further break up the flakes.

8. Add the half-and-half to the stockpot. Stir to combine. Cover the stockpot with the lid and heat the soup on low heat until it reaches serving temperature. Stir occasionally. Do not allow the soup to boil or the cream will separate. When the soup reaches serving temperature stir again to completely disperse the mashed potato flakes into the soup. Serve hot.

Jalapeno Chicken and Rice Stew

If you like the taste of jalapeno peppers then this dish will become a favorite. It uses prepared salsa verde (green salsa) and canned jalapenos for convenience and lots of lime, cumin, and oregano for flavor. Mellow Monterey Jack cheese tempers the heat of the jalapenos while the use of convenient frozen corn kernels helps to ensure that you get a serving of vegetables with your meal.

Ingredients

10 to 12 oz frozen corn kernels
2 TBSP vegetable oil
1 lb skinless boneless chicken breast, cut into 3/4" cubes
2 TBSP lime juice (about 2 limes)
1 4-oz can diced jalapeno peppers (do not drain)
1 24-oz jar salsa verde (green salsa)
2 TBSP dried onion flakes
1 1/2 tsp ground cumin
1 tsp granulated garlic *
1 1/2 tsp oregano, dried (use Mexican oregano for extra flavor)
2 cups long grain white rice
3 cups water
1 bunch cilantro, rinsed and finely minced
2 cups shredded Monterey Jack cheese * (about 8 oz by weight)

* See **Tips** section

Cookware and Utensils

6-quart stockpot with lid
Citrus juicer
Colander
Shredder/grater (if not using pre-shredded cheese)

Instructions

1. Transfer the frozen corn kernels to the countertop to thaw while you are preparing the other ingredients.

2. Add the oil to the stockpot. Cut the chicken into 3/4-inch cubes. Add the chicken to the stockpot. Stir to coat the chicken with the oil. Cover the stockpot with the lid. Cook the chicken on medium heat until it is completely cooked (opaque all the way through when cut with a knife). Stir occasionally.

3. While the chicken is cooking juice the limes.

4. When the chicken is fully cooked add the diced jalapeno peppers (do not drain), the salsa verde, and the lime juice to the stockpot. Stir to combine.

5. Add the onion flakes, cumin, garlic, and oregano to the stockpot. Stir to combine.

6. Add the rice to the stockpot. Stir to combine. Add 3 cups of water to the stockpot. Stir to combine. Cover the stockpot with the lid. Heat on medium high heat until the liquid boils then adjust the heat to a gentle simmer. Stir occasionally.

7. While the rice is cooking rinse the cilantro in the colander and allow it to drain thoroughly. Finely mince the leafy end of the cilantro bunch (discard the non-leafy stems). Add the minced cilantro to the stockpot. Stir to combine.

8. Shred the Monterey Jack cheese (if not using pre-shredded cheese).

9. When the water is almost all absorbed into the rice add the corn kernels to the stockpot. Stir to combine. Cover the stockpot with the lid and continue cooking, covered, until the rice is tender.

10. When the rice is completely cooked add the shredded Monterey Jack cheese to the stockpot. Stir to combine. Adjust the heat to medium low. Cover the stockpot with the lid and heat for a few minutes to melt the cheese.

11. When the cheese is fully melted stir again to evenly distribute the cheese into the rice. Serve immediately.

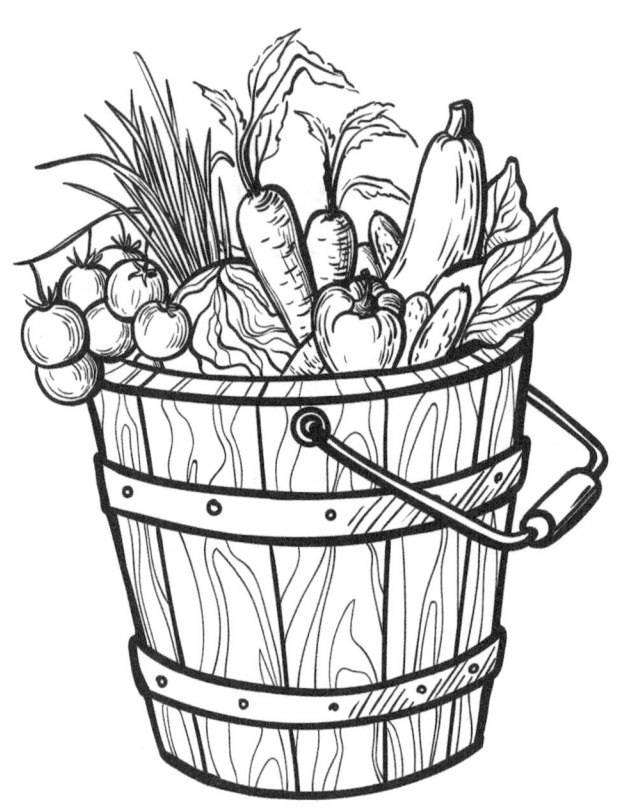

Pork

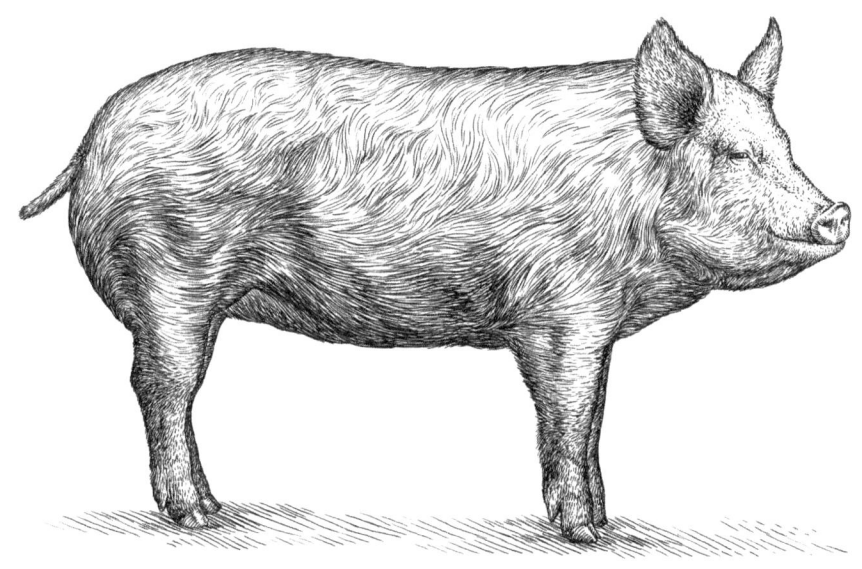

Meals in a Skillet

- 122 Creole Rice Skillet
- 123 Spanish Paella Skillet
- 124 Tastes Like Ravioli Skillet
- 125 Creamy Mushroom and Ham Skillet
- 126 Zesty Sausage, Potato, and Pepper Skillet
- 127 Hoppin' John
- 128 Skillet Red Beans and Rice with Spicy Sausage
- 130 Spanish Catalan Potato Skillet
- 131 Skillet Scalloped Potatoes and Ham with Mushrooms
- 132 Spaghetti Amatrice
- 133 Jammin' Jambalaya

Soups and Stews

- 134 Split Pea and Ham Soup
- 136 Winter Pork Stew with Smoked Paprika
- 138 Mexican Pork Chili Verde Stew
- 139 Italian White Bean, Ham, and Rosemary Soup
- 140 Spicy Sausage and Kale Soup
- 142 Fall Dinner Ham and Potato Soup
- 143 Easy French Cassoulet
- 144 Hearty Minestrone Soup in a Flash
- 146 Best Ever Pizza Soup
- 148 Tuscan Sausage and Bean Soup
- 150 Minnesota Wild Rice Soup
- 152 Spicy Chorizo Corn Chowder

Creole Rice Skillet

When asked to explain the difference between Creole and Cajun cooking one respondent declared 'Creole contains tomatoes, Cajun does not'. In truth there are additional subtle differences between these cuisines that figure prominently in the American South. Since this skillet contains tomatoes we will label it 'Creole'. The dish gets its flavor from smoked paprika and readily-available hot Italian sausage which is substituted for the traditional but harder-to-find Andouille sausage.

Ingredients

2 TBSP olive oil or vegetable oil
1 lb hot Italian sausage, in links *
1 cup onion chopped
   (about 1/2 of a large onion)
4 garlic cloves, chopped
1 red or green bell pepper,
   seeded and diced into 1/2" pieces
3 ribs celery,
   sliced into 3/8" thick slices
1 tsp salt
1 tsp oregano, dried
1 tsp thyme, dried
1/2 tsp black pepper
1/4 tsp hot red pepper flakes
1/4 tsp cayenne pepper
1 TBSP smoked paprika
1 15-oz can diced tomatoes
   (do not drain)
1 1/2 cups converted (parboiled) rice **
3 cups gluten-free chicken broth *
1 bay leaf
1 15-oz can red kidney beans,
   rinsed and drained

* See **Tips** section
** See **Converted Rice** section

Cookware and Utensils

12-inch skillet with lid
Cutting board
Small bowl
Colander

Instructions

1. Add the oil to the skillet. Arrange the sausages in an even layer on the bottom of the skillet. Pierce each sausage several times with the tines of a fork to allow juices to escape while cooking. Cover the skillet with the lid. Heat on medium low heat, turning the sausages once during cooking to brown both sides. Cook the sausages until they are no longer pink in the middle when cut with a knife.

2. While the sausages are cooking chop the onion. Chop the garlic. Seed the bell pepper. Dice the bell pepper into 1/2-inch pieces. Slice the celery into 3/8-inch thick slices.

3. When the sausages are done cooking transfer them to a cutting board. Skim excess fat from the pan drippings if desired, reserving a few tablespoons of drippings. Add the onion, garlic, bell pepper, and celery to the skillet. Stir to coat the vegetables with the sausage juices. Cook on medium heat until the onion is soft. Stir occasionally.

4. While the vegetables are cooking slice the sausages into 3/8-inch thick rounds.

5. Measure the salt, oregano, thyme, black pepper, red pepper flakes, cayenne pepper, and smoked paprika into a small bowl. Stir to combine. When the onion is soft add the seasonings to the vegetable mixture. Stir to coat the vegetables with the seasonings.

6. Add the tomatoes to the vegetable mixture (do not drain). Stir to combine. Add the converted (parboiled) rice to the vegetable mixture. Stir to coat the rice with the vegetables and seasonings. Add the sliced sausages to the rice and vegetable mixture. Stir to combine.

7. Add the chicken broth and the bay leaf to the rice and vegetable mixture. Stir to combine. Cover the skillet with the lid. Increase the heat to medium high until the mixture boils then reduce the heat to a gentle simmer. Stir occasionally.

8. While the rice is cooking rinse and drain the kidney beans in the colander. When the liquid is almost absorbed into the rice add the kidney beans to the skillet. Stir gently to combine.

9. When all of the liquid is fully absorbed into the rice remove the bay leaf. Serve immediately.

Spanish Paella Skillet

Paella (pie-AY-uh) is known as the national dish of Spain and has its roots in the regions around Barcelona. This easy skillet version of Spain's most famous dish gets its golden color from inexpensive turmeric instead of costly saffron. Readily-available hot Italian sausage substitutes for difficult-to-find dried Spanish chorizo while bottled clam juice adds seafood flavor. Add the optional shrimp for even better seafood flavor.

Ingredients

2 TBSP olive oil or vegetable oil
1 lb hot Italian sausage, in links *
1 cup onion chopped
  (about 1/2 of a large onion)
4 garlic cloves, chopped
1 red or green bell pepper,
  seeded and diced into 1/2" pieces
1 tsp salt
1 tsp turmeric
1/2 tsp oregano, dried
1/4 tsp black pepper
1 1/2 cups converted (parboiled) rice **
2 cups gluten-free chicken broth *
1 8-oz bottle clam juice *
1 bay leaf
8 to 10 oz pre-cooked frozen shrimp,
  peeled and deveined (optional)
1 cup frozen peas

* See *Tips* section
** See *Converted Rice* section

Cookware and Utensils

12-inch skillet with lid
Cutting board
Colander (if using the optional shrimp)

Instructions

1. Add the oil to the skillet. Arrange the sausages in an even layer on the bottom of the skillet. Pierce each sausage several times with the tines of a fork to allow juices to escape when cooking. Cover the skillet with the lid. Heat on medium low heat, turning the sausages once during cooking to brown both sides. Cook until the sausages are no longer pink in the middle when cut with a knife.

2. While the sausages are cooking chop the onion. Chop the garlic. Seed the bell pepper. Dice the bell pepper into 1/2-inch pieces.

3. When the sausages are done cooking transfer them to a cutting board. Skim excess fat from the skillet if desired. Add the onion, garlic, and bell pepper to the skillet. Stir to coat the vegetables with the sausage juices. Cook on medium heat until the onion is soft.

4. While the vegetables are cooking slice the sausages into 3/8-inch thick rounds.

5. When the onion is soft add the salt, turmeric, oregano, and black pepper to the vegetable mixture. Stir to coat the vegetables with the seasonings. Add the converted (parboiled) rice to the vegetable mixture. Stir to coat the rice with the vegetables and seasonings. Add the sliced sausages to the rice and vegetable mixture. Stir to combine.

6. Add the chicken broth, the clam juice, and the bay leaf to the rice and vegetable mixture. Stir to combine. Cover the skillet with the lid. Increase the heat to medium high until the mixture boils then reduce the heat to a gentle simmer. Stir occasionally.

7. While the rice is cooking rinse the (optional) frozen shrimp with cold water and drain.

8. When the liquid is almost absorbed into the rice add the peas and (optional) shrimp to the skillet. Stir gently to combine. Cook until all the liquid is absorbed into the rice and the (optional) shrimp is heated thoroughly. Remove the bay leaf. Serve immediately.

Tastes Like Ravioli Skillet

If you had to give up ravioli in a can when you went gluten-free you will be pleasantly surprised by this recipe that duplicates the flavors of the ravioli made famous by the Boy Chef.

Ingredients

1 lb mild Italian sausage *
1 cup onion, chopped
  (about 1/2 of a large onion)
1 tsp Italian seasoning
1/4 tsp hot red pepper flakes
1 24-oz jar spaghetti sauce
1 1/2 cups water, heated
8 oz gluten-free pasta **
2 cups shredded Mozzarella Cheese *
  (about 8 oz measured by weight)

* See *Tips* section
** See *Measuring Pasta* section

Cookware and Utensils

12-inch skillet with lid
Microwave-safe liquid measuring cup
  (2-cup size or larger)
Shredder/grater
  (if not using pre-shredded cheese)

Instructions

1. Remove the casings from the Italian sausage if necessary.

2. Add the Italian sausage to the skillet, breaking it into small chunks, about 3/4-inch in size. Cover the skillet with the lid. Brown the sausage on medium heat.

3. While the sausage is browning chop the onion.

4. Check the sausage for doneness. The sausage is fully cooked when there is no pink color. Drain the fat from the sausage.

5. Add the chopped onion, Italian seasoning, and red pepper flakes to the sausage. Continue cooking on medium heat, stirring occasionally, until the onion is soft.

6. When the onion is soft add the spaghetti sauce to the sausage mixture. Stir to combine.

7. Microwave 1 1/2 cups of water on high power for 2 minutes. Add the hot water to the sausage mixture. Stir to combine.

8. Add the gluten-free pasta to the sausage mixture. Stir to combine. Cover the skillet with the lid. Increase the heat to medium high until the mixture boils then reduce the heat to a gentle simmer.

9. Stir the mixture frequently, checking every 3 to 4 minutes until the pasta is cooked to your taste. It will take longer for the pasta to cook in this recipe because of the tomato sauce in the cooking liquid.

10. While the pasta is cooking shred the Mozzarella cheese (if not using pre-shredded cheese).

11. When the pasta is cooked to the desired doneness sprinkle the Mozzarella cheese over the top of the skillet. Turn off the heat and cover the skillet with the lid. Allow the cheese to fully melt. Serve immediately.

Creamy Mushroom and Ham Skillet

This quick and easy ham and mushroom skillet is perfect for a night when you don't have a lot of time to make dinner. If you don't like peas then substitute frozen broccoli florets (2 cups) or frozen cut green beans (1 cup).

Ingredients

1/2 cup onion, finely chopped
3 TBSP butter
8 oz white button mushrooms, washed and sliced
8 oz ham, diced into 3/8" cubes *
1 cup water, heated
1 tsp salt
1/2 tsp thyme, dried
1/2 tsp granulated garlic *
1/4 tsp black pepper
2 cups milk *
8 oz gluten-free pasta **
3/4 cup grated Parmesan cheese *
1 cup frozen peas

* See *Tips* section
** See *Measuring Pasta* section

Cookware and Utensils

12-inch skillet with lid
Colander
Microwave-safe liquid measuring cup (1-cup size or larger)
Shredder/grater (if not using pre-grated cheese)

Instructions

1. Finely chop the onion.

2. Add the butter and the onion to the skillet. Heat on low heat until the onion is soft, stirring frequently.

3. Rinse the mushrooms in the colander and allow them to drain. Slice the mushrooms. Add the mushrooms to the onion mixture. Stir to combine. Cover the skillet with the lid. Increase the heat to medium. Stir occasionally.

4. Dice the ham into 3/8-inch cubes. Add the ham to the mushroom and onion mixture. Stir to combine.

5. Microwave 1 cup of water on high power for 1 minute.

6. When the mushrooms are soft add the salt, thyme, garlic, and black pepper to the skillet. Stir to combine.

7. Add the hot water and the milk to the skillet. Stir to combine.

8. Add the gluten-free pasta to the skillet. Stir to combine. Cover the skillet with the lid. Increase the heat to medium high until the mixture boils then reduce the heat to a gentle simmer.

9. Most gluten-free pastas cook in 7 to 12 minutes. Stir the mixture frequently, checking every 3 to 4 minutes until the pasta is cooked to your taste.

10. While the pasta is cooking grate the Parmesan cheese (if not using pre-grated cheese).

11. When the pasta is cooked to the desired doneness stir in the frozen peas or alternate vegetable. Cover the skillet with the lid and heat until the vegetables are tender crisp.

12. Stir in the grated Parmesan cheese. Cover the skillet with the lid. Reduce the heat to low and heat for a few minutes to melt the cheese. When the cheese is fully melted stir again to fully combine the cheese. Serve immediately.

Zesty Sausage, Potato, and Pepper Skillet

This skillet dinner evokes a bygone era when farm families sat down to a hearty meal of simple ingredients - a skillet of sausages, potatoes, savory onions, and peppers. You can use mild Italian sausage in this recipe or substitute hot Italian sausage if you like your food spicy.

Ingredients

3 TBSP olive oil or vegetable oil
12 to 16 oz mild or hot Italian sausage, in links *
1 large onion, sliced into crescents
3 cloves garlic, chopped
1 red bell pepper, seeded and diced into 1/2" pieces
1 green bell pepper, seeded and diced into 1/2" pieces
1/2 tsp salt
1/2 tsp black pepper
1 1/2 tsp Hungarian Sweet Paprika (substitute regular paprika)
28-oz or 32-oz package frozen diced hash brown potatoes
(frozen cubed potatoes)

* See *Tips* section

Cookware and Utensils

12-inch skillet with lid
Cutting board
Spatula

Instructions

1. Add the oil to the skillet.

2. Arrange the sausages in an even layer on the bottom of the skillet. Pierce each sausage several times with the tines of a fork to release juices while cooking. Cover the skillet with the lid. Cook the sausages on medium low heat until they are fully cooked (no pink color when sliced open). Turn once during cooking to brown both sides of the sausages.

3. While the sausages are cooking slice the onion into crescents.

4. Chop the garlic.

5. Wash and seed the bell peppers. Dice the bell peppers into 1/2-inch pieces.

6. When the sausages are done cooking transfer them to a cutting board to cool. Add the onion, garlic, and the bell peppers to the skillet. Stir to coat the vegetables with the sausage juices. Increase the heat to medium and cook, uncovered, until the onion is soft. Stir occasionally.

7. While the vegetables are cooking slice the sausages into 3/8-inch thick rounds. When the onion is soft add the sliced sausages to the skillet. Stir to combine.

8. Sprinkle the salt, pepper, and paprika on the vegetable and sausage mixture. Stir to coat the vegetables and the sausage with the seasonings.

9. Add the frozen diced hash brown potatoes to the skillet. Stir to combine. Increase the heat to medium high and cook, uncovered, until the bottom of the potatoes develops a golden crust.

10. Use the spatula to flip the potato mixture. Continue cooking, uncovered, on medium high heat until the potatoes are browned on the bottom. Serve immediately.

Hoppin' John

Hoppin' John is a dish consisting of black-eyed peas and rice that is traditionally served on New Year's Day. Originating from African, French, and Caribbean roots it is believed to bring a prosperous year filled with good luck. The black-eyed peas are symbolic of coins and some cooks place a coin under one of the dinner plates. The lucky recipient of the coin is said to receive the most good luck in the coming year. This easy one-pot version of the dish combines the rice and black-eyed peas for convenience.

Ingredients

6 slices thick-cut bacon,
  diced into 1/2" pieces (about 8 oz)
12 oz ham, diced into 1/2" cubes *
  (optional)
1 1/2 cups onion, chopped
6 cloves garlic, chopped
1 green bell pepper,
  seeded and diced into 1/2" pieces
3 ribs celery, ends trimmed,
  sliced into 3/8" thick slices
3/4 tsp salt
1/2 tsp black pepper
1/2 tsp thyme, dried
1/2 tsp basil, dried
1 tsp oregano, dried
1/2 tsp cayenne pepper
1 2/3 cups long-grain white rice
1 quart gluten-free chicken broth
  or ham broth *
2 TBSP apple cider vinegar
2 bay leaves
2 15-oz cans black-eyed peas,
  rinsed and drained

* See *Tips* section

Cookware and Utensils

6-quart stockpot with lid
Small bowl for seasonings
Small heatproof bowl
Colander

Instructions

1. Cut the bacon into 1/2-inch pieces. Add the bacon to the stockpot. Crisp the bacon on medium heat, stirring frequently. If you will be adding the (optional) ham then dice it into 1/2-inch cubes.

2. While the bacon is crisping chop the onion and the garlic. Wash and seed the bell pepper. Dice the bell pepper into 1/2-inch pieces. Trim the ends of the celery ribs and slice them into 3/8-inch thick slices.

3. Add the salt, black pepper, thyme, basil, oregano, and cayenne pepper to the small bowl. Stir to combine.

4. When the bacon is crisp drain some of the grease by moving the stockpot to an unused burner, tipping it away from you, and carefully spooning the hot grease into a small heatproof bowl. Reserve about 3 tablespoons of bacon drippings in the stockpot. Allow the hot grease to cool before disposing. Return the stockpot to the heated burner. Add the onion, garlic, bell pepper, celery, and (optional) diced ham to the stockpot. Stir to combine. Cover the stockpot with the lid and cook on medium heat until the onion is soft.

5. When the onion is soft add the seasonings to the bacon and vegetable mixture. Stir to coat the vegetables with the seasonings. Add the rice to the stockpot. Stir to coat the rice with the vegetables and seasonings.

6. Add the chicken broth and the apple cider vinegar to the stockpot. Stir to combine.

7. Add the bay leaves to the stockpot, submerging them below the broth. Cover the stockpot with the lid. Increase the heat to medium high until the mixture boils then reduce the heat to a gentle simmer. Simmer, covered, until the rice is fully cooked. Do not stir.

8. While the rice is cooking rinse and drain the black-eyed peas in the colander. When the rice is tender and has absorbed all of the liquid remove the bay leaves. Gently stir in the black-eyed peas. Cover the stockpot with the lid. Reduce the heat to low and heat for a few minutes to warm the black-eyed peas. Serve immediately.

Skillet Red Beans and Rice with Spicy Sausage

Red Beans and Rice is a New Orleans tradition which is commonly served as a bean and sausage porridge over a bed of white rice. This skillet version combines the beans, sausage, and rice together in one pan for convenience and quick time to table.

Ingredients

2 TBSP olive oil or vegetable oil
12 to 16 oz Andouille, Cajun,
  or hot Italian sausage, in links *
1 1/2 cups onion, chopped
1 green bell pepper,
  seeded and diced into 1/2" pieces
3 ribs celery, sliced into 3/8" thick slices
1 tsp salt
1/2 tsp black pepper
1 tsp thyme, dried
1 tsp oregano, dried
1 tsp paprika
1/2 tsp cayenne pepper
1 1/2 tsp granulated garlic *
1 1/3 cups long grain white rice
3 cups gluten-free chicken broth *
2 bay leaves
2 15-oz cans kidney beans,
  rinsed and drained

* See **Tips** section

Instructions

1. Add the oil to the skillet. Arrange the sausages in an even layer on the bottom of the skillet. Pierce each sausage several times with the tines of a fork to allow juices to escape while cooking. Cover the skillet with the lid. Heat on medium low heat, turning the sausages once during cooking to brown both sides. Cook the sausages until they are no longer pink in the middle when cut with a knife.

2. While the sausages are cooking chop the onion. Dice the bell pepper into 1/2-inch pieces. Slice the celery into 3/8-inch thick slices.

3. Measure the salt, black pepper, thyme, oregano, paprika, cayenne pepper, and garlic into the small bowl. Stir to combine the seasonings.

4. When the sausages are done cooking transfer them to a cutting board. Skim excess fat from the pan drippings, reserving a few tablespoons of drippings. Add the onion, bell pepper, and celery to the skillet. Stir to coat the vegetables with the sausage juices. Cook on medium heat until the onion is soft. Stir occasionally.

5. While the vegetables are cooking slice the sausages into 3/8-inch thick rounds.

6. When the onion is soft add the seasonings to the vegetable mixture. Stir to coat the vegetables with the seasonings.

7. Add the rice to the vegetable mixture. Stir to coat the rice with the vegetables and seasonings.

8. Add the sliced sausages to the skillet. Stir to combine.

9. Add the chicken broth to the skillet. Stir to combine.

10. Add the bay leaves and submerge them below the broth. Cover the skillet with the lid. Increase the heat to medium high until the broth boils then reduce the heat to a gentle simmer. Keep the lid on the skillet and do not stir while the rice is cooking.

Continued

Skillet Red Beans and Rice with Spicy Sausage

- Continued -

Cookware and Utensils

12-inch skillet with lid
Small bowl
Cutting board
Colander

Instructions - continued

11. While the rice is cooking rinse the kidney beans in the colander and allow them to drain thoroughly.

12. When the liquid is almost absorbed into the rice add the drained kidney beans to the skillet. Stir gently to combine. Cover the skillet with the lid. Reduce the heat to low and continue cooking until all the liquid is absorbed into the rice.

13. When all of the liquid is absorbed into the rice remove the bay leaves. Serve immediately.

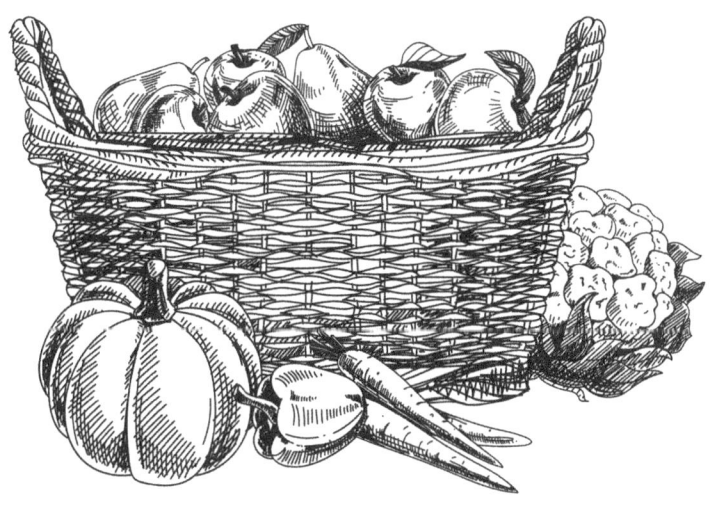

Spanish Catalan Potato Skillet

Catalonia is a region of Spain that encompasses Barcelona, bordering France and the Mediterranean Sea. The region is well known for its paella, tapas, and flavorful hams. This recipe is a variation of Patatas Aborregas (Shepherd's Potatoes) featuring the abundant ham and tomatoes found in the region. This simple peasant dish is seasoned with Smoked Paprika which lends a heady flavor of bacon.

Ingredients

2 lbs potatoes, scrubbed, halved lengthwise, and sliced thinly into 3/8" thick slices
3 cups water
2 cups onion, sliced into crescents
4 cloves garlic, chopped
12 oz ham, diced into 1/2" cubes *
1 pint cherry tomatoes, rinsed and cut in half
3/4 tsp salt
1/2 tsp black pepper
2 tsp smoked paprika
1/4 tsp thyme, dried
1 tsp rosemary, dried
3 TBSP olive oil or vegetable oil

* See *Tips* section

Cookware and Utensils

12-inch skillet with lid
Small bowl
Spatula

Instructions

1. Scrub the potatoes under running water. Slice the potatoes in half lengthwise. Cut each potato half into 3/8-inch thick slices. Layer the potato slices on the bottom of the skillet.

2. Pour the water into the skillet. Cover the skillet with the lid. Cook on medium high heat until the water begins to boil then adjust the heat to a gentle simmer. Cook the potatoes until they just begin to get tender but are not completely cooked (about 8 minutes). Leave the lid on the skillet during cooking and do not stir.

3. While the potatoes are cooking slice the onion into crescents.

4. Chop the garlic.

5. Dice the ham into 1/2-inch cubes.

6. Rinse the cherry tomatoes and slice them in half.

7. Add the salt, pepper, smoked paprika, thyme, and rosemary to the small bowl. Stir to combine.

8. When the potatoes are just beginning to get tender drain the water from the skillet. Drizzle the oil over the potatoes. Add the onion, garlic, and the ham to the skillet. Use a spatula to gently combine the potatoes, oil, ham, and vegetables, taking care not to break up the potato slices.

9. Use the spatula to press down on the potato mixture to flatten it. Sprinkle the mixed seasonings over the potatoes. Cover the skillet with the lid. Increase the heat to medium high and cook, covered, until the potatoes form a golden crust on the bottom.

10. When the bottom side of the potatoes has browned use the spatula to flip the potatoes. Layer the halved cherry tomatoes over the potatoes. Use the spatula to press the tomatoes into the potatoes. Cover the skillet with the lid. Reduce the heat to medium and continue cooking, covered, until the onion is soft and the tomatoes begin to soften.

11. When the onion is soft remove the lid from the skillet. Cook, uncovered, until a golden crust forms on the bottom of the potatoes. Serve hot.

Skillet Scalloped Potatoes and Ham with Mushrooms

Sometimes you crave the taste of scalloped potatoes and ham but you don't want to turn on the oven. This quick and easy skillet version is on the table fast with only one pan to clean up.

Ingredients

32 oz unflavored frozen diced hash brown potatoes (frozen cubed potatoes)
4 TBSP butter
1 cup onion, chopped
 (about 1/2 of a large onion)
12 oz ham, diced into 3/8" cubes *
8 oz mushrooms, washed and sliced
1/2 tsp salt
1/2 tsp black pepper
1 tsp granulated garlic *
8 oz sour cream *
1 1/2 cups half-and-half
1 cup grated Parmesan cheese *

* See *Tips* section

Cookware and Utensils

12-inch skillet with lid
Colander
Shredder/grater
 (if not using pre-grated cheese)

Instructions

1. Transfer the frozen diced hash brown potatoes to the countertop to thaw while you prepare the other ingredients.

2. Add the butter to the skillet. Melt the butter on low heat.

3. While the butter is melting chop the onion. Add the onion to the skillet. Increase the heat to medium low and cook, stirring occasionally, until the onion is soft.

4. While the onion is cooking dice the ham into 3/8-inch cubes.

5. Rinse and drain the mushrooms in the colander. Slice the mushrooms.

6. When the onion is soft add the diced ham to the skillet. Stir to combine.

7. Add the salt, pepper, and garlic to the skillet. Stir to combine.

8. Add the mushrooms to the skillet. Stir to combine. Cover the skillet with the lid. Increase the heat to medium and cook, covered, until the mushrooms are soft.

9. When the mushrooms are soft add the sour cream to the skillet. Stir to combine.

10. Add the half-and-half to the skillet. Stir to combine.

11. Add the hash brown potatoes to the skillet. Stir to combine. Cover the skillet with the lid and increase the heat to medium high until the potatoes begin to simmer. Reduce the heat to maintain a gentle simmer. Cook, covered, until the potatoes are tender. Do not overcook or the potatoes will become mushy.

12. While the potatoes are cooking grate the Parmesan cheese (if not using pre-grated cheese).

13. When the potatoes are tender add the Parmesan cheese to the skillet. Stir gently to combine. Cover the skillet with the lid and turn off the heat. Wait a few minutes for the cheese to melt, then stir gently again to combine the cheese into the potatoes. Serve immediately.

Spaghetti Amatrice

In the heart of Italy lies the small village of Amatrice which is famous for its pasta dishes so delicious that many chefs from this tiny hamlet were asked to come to Rome to cook for the Popes. Our easy version of Spaghetti Amatrice substitutes thick cut bacon for the traditional Guanciale which is a cured seasoned pig's jowl that is difficult to find outside of Italy. Readily available Parmesan cheese substitutes for the traditional but expensive sheep's milk Pecorino Romano cheese.

Ingredients

6 slices thick cut bacon,
  diced into 1/2" pieces
2 TBSP dried onion flakes
1/2 tsp salt
1/4 tsp black pepper
1/2 tsp rosemary, dried
1/2 tsp basil, dried
  (substitute 1 TBSP fresh chopped basil)
1/2 tsp oregano, dried
1/2 tsp hot red pepper flakes
1 28-oz can tomatoes, diced or crushed
  (do not drain)
2 TBSP olive oil
1/2 cup white wine (substitute water)
3 cups water
12 oz corn and rice blend
  gluten-free spaghetti **
2/3 cup grated Parmesan cheese *

* See *Tips* section
** Use only gluten-free spaghetti that is made from a corn and rice blend. The corn will keep the spaghetti from becoming gummy as it cooks.

Cookware and Utensils

12-inch skillet with lid
Small bowl
Metal mesh sieve
Small heatproof bowl
Shredder/grater
  (if not using pre-grated cheese)

Instructions

1. Dice the bacon into 1/2-inch pieces. Add the bacon to the skillet. Crisp the bacon on medium heat, stirring frequently.

2. While the bacon is crisping add the onion flakes, salt, pepper, rosemary, dried basil, oregano, and red pepper flakes to the small bowl. Stir to combine. Set aside. If you are substituting fresh basil chop it coarsely and set it aside.

3. When the bacon is crisp position the metal mesh sieve over the heatproof bowl. Pour the bacon and drippings into the sieve and allow the bacon to drain thoroughly. When the bacon is well-drained return it to the skillet. Allow the bacon grease to cool before disposing.

4. Add the tomatoes (do not drain), olive oil, white wine (substitute water), and 3 cups of water to the skillet. Stir to combine.

5. Add the mixed seasonings (and the fresh basil if you are using it) to the skillet. Stir to combine. Cover the skillet with the lid. Increase the heat to medium high until the tomato mixture boils.

6. Break the spaghetti in half. When the tomato mixture is boiling add the spaghetti to the skillet in a crisscross pattern, a few strands at a time, distributing it evenly to keep the spaghetti strands from sticking to each other. Use a large-bowl spoon to scoop the sauce over the spaghetti to moisten and submerge the spaghetti in the sauce.

7. After the spaghetti begins to soften use a fork to gently separate any strands that have stuck together. Cover the skillet with the lid. Adjust the heat to a gentle simmer. Stir occasionally, cooking until the spaghetti is 'al dente' (soft but with 'a bite').

8. While the spaghetti is cooking grate the Parmesan cheese (if not using pre-grated cheese). When the spaghetti is cooked to your taste sprinkle the grated cheese over the skillet. Stir gently to combine. Cover the skillet with the lid. Turn off the heat and allow the cheese to melt. Stir again to evenly distribute the cheese throughout the dish. Serve immediately.

Jammin' Jambalaya

New Orleans is known for both its jazz music and its Cajun and Creole cooking brought to the Louisiana delta by French and Spanish settlers. The New Orleans version of Spanish paella is Jambalaya which uses the delta's plentiful shrimp, ham, and flavorful Andouille sausage. If you can't find Andouille sausage at your market then substitute Cajun sausage or readily available hot Italian sausage.

Ingredients

2 TBSP olive oil (substitute vegetable oil)
8 to 12 oz Andouille, Cajun,
  or hot Italian sausage, in links *
1 cup onion, chopped
  (about 1/2 of a large onion)
4 cloves garlic, chopped
1 green or red bell pepper, seeded and
  diced into 1/2" pieces
3 ribs celery, sliced thinly
  into 3/8" thick slices
8 oz ham, diced into 1/2" cubes *
1 tsp salt
1/2 tsp black pepper
1 tsp thyme, dried
1 tsp oregano, dried
1/2 tsp basil, dried
1/2 tsp hot red pepper flakes
1/2 tsp paprika
1/2 tsp cayenne pepper
1 1/2 cups converted (parboiled) rice **
1 15-oz can crushed or diced tomatoes
  (do not drain)
3 cups gluten-free ham broth *
  (substitute gluten-free chicken broth)
1 bay leaf
4 oz frozen pre-cooked and peeled
  bay shrimp (salad shrimp)
* See *Tips* section
** See *Converted Rice* section

Cookware and Utensils

12-inch skillet with lid
Small bowl
Cutting board
Colander

Instructions

1. Add the oil and the sausages to the skillet. Heat on medium low heat, turning the sausages once during cooking to brown both sides. Cook the sausages until they are no longer pink in the middle. While the sausages are cooking chop the onion, garlic, and bell pepper. Slice the celery into 3/8-inch thick slices. Dice the ham into 1/2-inch cubes.

2. Measure the salt, black pepper, thyme, oregano, basil, red pepper flakes, paprika, and cayenne pepper into the small bowl. Stir to combine the seasonings.

3. When the sausages are done cooking transfer them to a cutting board. Skim excess fat from the pan drippings if desired, reserving a few tablespoons of drippings. Add the onion, garlic, bell pepper, celery, and diced ham to the skillet. Stir to coat the vegetables with the sausage juices. Cook on medium heat until the onion is soft. Stir occasionally.

4. While the ham and vegetables are cooking slice the sausages into 3/8-inch thick rounds. When the onion is soft add the seasonings to the vegetable mixture. Stir to coat the vegetables with the seasonings. Add the converted (parboiled) rice to the vegetable mixture. Stir to coat the rice with the vegetables and seasonings. Add the sliced sausages and the canned tomatoes (do not drain) to the rice and vegetable mixture. Stir to combine.

5. Add the ham broth or chicken broth to the rice and vegetable mixture. Stir to combine. Add the bay leaf and submerge it below the broth. Cover the skillet with the lid. Increase the heat to medium high until the mixture boils then reduce the heat to a gentle simmer. Stir occasionally.

6. While the rice is cooking thaw the frozen shrimp by rinsing it with cold water in the colander. Allow the shrimp to drain thoroughly.

7. When the liquid is almost absorbed into the rice add the drained shrimp to the skillet. Stir gently to combine. Cover the skillet with the lid. Continue cooking until all the liquid is fully absorbed into the rice. Remove the bay leaf. Serve immediately.

Split Pea and Ham Soup

Peas were a plentiful high-protein, low-cost food in ancient England, Europe, and Scandinavia so it's no surprise that the Brits, Germans, Poles, Swedes, and the Fins all have their own version of Split Pea and Ham Soup. Serve this soup with the optional garlic croutons if desired.

Ingredients

1 quart gluten-free chicken broth *
1 cup split peas, dry (about 8 oz)
12 oz ham, diced into 1/2" cubes *
1 cup onion, chopped
  (about 1/2 of a large onion)
1 tsp salt
1/2 tsp black pepper
1/2 tsp marjoram, dried
1/4 tsp thyme, dried
1 bay leaf
4 carrots, ends trimmed,
  sliced in half lengthwise,
  halves sliced into 3/8" thick slices
4 celery ribs, ends trimmed,
  sliced in half lengthwise,
  halves sliced into 3/8" thick slices

Optional Croutons

8 slices gluten-free bread
2 TBSP olive oil
2 tsp granulated garlic *

* See **Tips** section

Instructions

1. If you will be making the (optional) garlic croutons then preheat the oven to 300 degrees F.

2. Add the chicken broth to the stockpot. Cover the stockpot with the lid. Heat on medium high heat until the broth begins to boil then reduce the heat to a gentle simmer.

3. Transfer the peas to the mesh sieve. Rinse and drain the peas thoroughly. Inspect the peas for rocks or other foreign matter that could chip a tooth and discard if necessary. Add the drained peas to the stockpot. Stir to combine.

4. Dice the ham into 1/2-inch cubes. Add the ham to the stockpot. Stir to combine.

5. Chop the onion and add it to the stockpot. Stir to combine.

6. Add the salt, pepper, marjoram, thyme, and the bay leaf to the stockpot. Stir to combine. Cover the stockpot with the lid. Adjust the heat until the broth simmers gently. Stir occasionally.

7. If you will be making the (optional) garlic croutons then line a baking sheet with aluminum foil or parchment paper. Cut each piece of gluten-free bread into four squares. Arrange the squares of bread in a single layer on the lined baking sheet.

8. Transfer the baking sheet to the preheated oven. Toast the first side of the bread squares until slightly crunchy (about 10 minutes).

9. While the croutons are toasting scrub the carrots under running water and trim their ends. Slice each carrot in half lengthwise then slice the halves into 3/8-inch thick slices.

10. Wash the celery ribs and trim their ends. Slice each rib in half lengthwise then slice the halves into 3/8-inch thick slices.

Continued

Split Pea and Ham Soup
- Continued -

Cookware and Utensils

6-quart stockpot with lid
Mesh sieve
Metal baking sheet (optional)
Aluminum foil or parchment paper (optional)
Basting brush (optional)

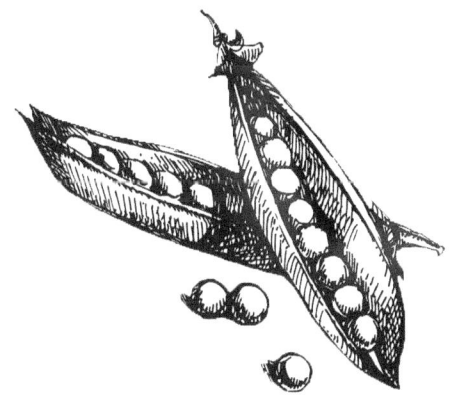

Instructions - continued

11. After the first side of the bread squares has been toasted remove the baking sheet from the oven. Flip each bread square. Baste the top side of the bread squares with 2 tablespoons of olive oil. Sprinkle the bread squares lightly with 2 teaspoons of granulated garlic. Return the baking sheet to the oven. Toast the bread squares until golden brown (about 10 minutes). Turn off the oven and keep the croutons warm in the oven until serving time.

12. After the soup has simmered for 20 minutes add the celery and carrots to the stockpot. Stir to combine. Cover the stockpot with the lid. Increase the heat to medium high until the soup begins to boil again then reduce the heat to a gentle simmer. Continue to simmer the soup, covered, for another 30 minutes. Stir occasionally.

13. After the soup has simmered for the additional 30 minutes test for doneness. The soup is done when the peas are tender. If you prefer your soup creamy you can continue to simmer the soup until the peas break down completely.

14. Remove the bay leaf before serving. Serve the soup hot with (optional) warm garlic croutons.

Winter Pork Stew with Smoked Paprika

On a cold winter night nothing satisfies like a hot steaming bowl of stew. This hearty pork stew gets its heat from a generous measure of smoked paprika that warms both the tongue and the tummy. Unlike the relatively bland paprika you may be used to cooking with, smoked paprika has a savory, dense flavor with hints of wood-smoked bacon. This dish tastes even better the next day so save the leftovers for a delicious lunch.

Ingredients

2 TBSP vegetable oil
1 1/2 lbs boneless pork shoulder,
  cut into 3/4" cubes
2 cups onion, chopped
  (about 1 large onion)
8 oz white button mushrooms,
  washed and sliced
1 1/2 tsp salt
1/4 tsp black pepper
1/4 tsp caraway seed
1 tsp thyme, dried
2 tsp granulated garlic *
2 TBSP smoked paprika
1 8-oz can tomato sauce
1 cup red wine
3 cups gluten-free beef broth *
  (reserve 1 cup)
1 tsp apple cider vinegar
1 lb carrots, ends trimmed,
  cut into 1" lengths
1 lb potatoes, cut into 1" cubes
1/4 cup cornstarch

* See **Tips** section

Optional Warm Buttered Bread
8 slices gluten-free bread
3 TBSP butter

Instructions

1. If you will be making the (optional) warm buttered bread then preheat the oven to 200 degrees F. Butter one side of each slice of gluten-free bread. Assemble the slices into a loaf. Wrap the loaf with aluminum foil. Transfer the foil-wrapped loaf into the preheated oven.

2. Add the oil to the stockpot.

3. Trim excess fat from the pork and cut it into 3/4-inch cubes. Add the pork to the stockpot. Stir to coat the pork with the oil. Brown the pork on medium heat, stirring occasionally.

4. While the pork is browning chop the onion. When the pork is brown add the onion to the stockpot. Stir to combine. Reduce the heat to medium low and cook, stirring occasionally, until the onion is soft.

5. Rinse the mushrooms in the colander and allow them to drain thoroughly. Slice the mushrooms. When the onion is soft add the mushrooms to the stockpot. Stir to combine. Cover the stockpot with the lid and cook until the mushrooms are soft.

6. Add the salt, pepper, caraway seed, thyme, garlic, and smoked paprika to the small bowl. Stir to combine.

7. When the mushrooms are soft add the mixed seasonings to the stockpot. Stir to coat the pork and vegetables with the seasonings.

8. Add the tomato sauce to the stockpot. Stir to combine.

9. Add the red wine, 2 cups of the beef broth, and the apple cider vinegar to the stockpot. Stir to combine. Cover the stockpot with the lid. Increase the heat to medium high until the mixture boils then reduce the heat to a gentle simmer.

10. Scrub the carrots under running water and trim their ends. Slice the carrots into 1-inch lengths. Add the carrots to the stockpot. Stir to combine.

Continued

Winter Pork Stew with Smoked Paprika
- Continued -

Cookware and Utensils

6-quart stockpot with lid
Colander
Small bowl
2-cup liquid measuring cup
Aluminum foil (optional)

Instructions - continued

11. Scrub the potatoes under running water. Cut the potatoes into 1-inch cubes. Add the potatoes to the stockpot. Stir to combine. Cover the stockpot with the lid. Increase the heat to medium high until the stew begins to boil then reduce the heat to a gentle simmer.

12. Transfer the reserved cup of beef broth to the liquid measuring cup. Add the cornstarch to the beef broth. Use a fork to mix the broth and break up any clumps. Stir until the cornstarch is completely dissolved into the broth.

13. Slowly add the broth and cornstarch mixture to the stockpot, stirring the stew continuously to avoid clumping of the cornstarch. Cover the stockpot with the lid. Adjust the heat until the stew comes to a gentle simmer. Simmer the stew until the potatoes and carrots pierce easily with the tines of a fork.

14. When the vegetables are tender the stew is done. Serve the stew hot with the (optional) warm buttered bread.

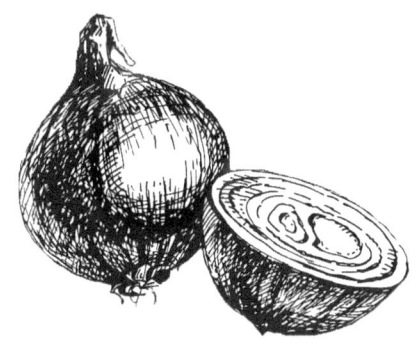

Mexican Pork Chili Verde Stew

Traditional Chili Verde ('green chili') is made with tomatillos which are green tomato-like fruits that are enclosed in a papery husk. The preparation of Chili Verde can be an all-day affair in which the tomatillos are slow-simmered with fire roasted chili peppers and hunks of pork shoulder meat. This hybrid between traditional Chili Verde and the stews of the American Southwest makes use of readily-available Salsa Verde ('green salsa') and canned peppers so you don't have to spend all day in the kitchen.

Ingredients

2 TBSP vegetable oil
1 1/2 lbs boneless pork shoulder, cut into 3/4" cubes
2 cups red onion, sliced into crescents
1 bell pepper (red, green, or yellow), seeded and diced into 1/2" pieces
1 24-oz jar salsa verde (green salsa)
1 4-oz can diced mild green chilis (do not drain)
1 4-oz can diced jalapeno peppers, measure 1 tablespoon, add more to taste if desired
1 1/2 tsp oregano, dried
1/2 tsp salt
2 tsp ground cumin
1 TBSP granulated garlic *
1 lb carrots, cut into 1" lengths
1 1/2 lbs potatoes, cut into 1" cubes
3 TBSP lime juice (2-3 limes)
1 bunch cilantro, destemmed, leaves coarsely chopped

* See **Tips** section

Cookware and Utensils

6-quart stockpot with lid
Citrus juicer

Instructions

1. Add the oil to the stockpot. Cut the pork into 3/4-inch cubes. Add the pork to the stockpot. Brown the pork on medium heat, stirring occasionally.

2. While the pork is browning slice the red onion into crescents. Seed and dice the bell pepper into 1/2-inch pieces.

3. When the pork has browned add the red onion and bell pepper to the stockpot. Stir to combine. Continue cooking on medium heat, stirring occasionally, until the onion is soft.

4. When the onion is soft add the salsa verde to the stockpot. Stir to combine. Add the green chilis (do not drain) and one tablespoon of the diced jalapeno peppers to the stockpot. Stir to combine.

5. Add the oregano, salt, cumin, and garlic to the stockpot. Stir to combine.

6. Scrub and trim the ends of the carrots. Cut the carrots into 1-inch lengths. Add the carrots to the stockpot. Stir to combine.

7. Scrub the potatoes under running water. You may peel the potatoes if desired. Cut the potatoes into 1-inch cubes. Add the potatoes to the stockpot. Stir to combine. Cover the stockpot with the lid. Increase the heat to medium high until the stew boils then reduce the heat to a gentle simmer. Simmer the stew covered, stirring occasionally, until the carrots and potatoes pierce easily with the tines of a fork.

8. While the stew is simmering juice the limes.

9. Wash and destem the cilantro. Coarsely chop the cilantro leaves.

10. When the carrots and potatoes are tender add the lime juice and the cilantro to the stockpot. Stir to combine.

11. Taste the stew for flavor balance. If you like your stew spicy then add additional diced jalapeno pepper in one tablespoon increments until it is spicy enough for your taste. Stir to combine. Store unused jalapeno pepper in a plastic or glass container in your freezer for up to a month. Serve the stew hot.

Italian White Bean, Ham, and Rosemary Soup

In Italy, Zuppa di Fagioli (Bean Soup) is a traditional meal. This quick and easy version of the traditional Italian favorite gets its unique flavor from a combination of rosemary, thyme, sage, and a dash of hot red pepper flakes. You can use any type of white beans - Great Northern, Navy, or Cannellini - or try a combination. Serve this soup topped with grated Parmesan cheese and the (optional) warm gluten-free bread.

Ingredients

2 cups onion, chopped
  (about 1 large onion)
3 TBSP olive oil or vegetable oil
1 tsp rosemary, dried
  (substitute 1 TBSP fresh rosemary)
1/4 tsp thyme, dried
  (substitute 1 tsp fresh thyme leaves)
1/4 tsp ground sage
  (substitute 1 tsp fresh sage leaves)
1 1/4 tsp salt
1/4 tsp black pepper
1/4 tsp hot red pepper flakes
1 1/2 tsp granulated garlic *
12 oz ham, diced into 1/2" cubes *
1 quart gluten-free chicken broth
  or ham broth *
1 bay leaf
2 carrots, ends trimmed,
  halved lengthwise,
  halves sliced into 3/8" thick slices
2 ribs celery, ends trimmed,
  halved lengthwise,
  halves sliced into 3/8" thick slices
2 15-oz cans white beans (Cannellini,
  Great Northern, Navy, or other white
  beans), rinsed and drained
1/4 cup grated Parmesan cheese *
* See **Tips** section

Optional Warm Gluten-Free Bread
8 slices gluten-free bread

Cookware and Utensils

6-quart stockpot with lid
Colander   Shredder/grater
Small serving bowl
Aluminum foil (optional)

Instructions

1. If you will be making the (optional) warm gluten-free bread then preheat the oven to 200 degrees F. Assemble the slices of gluten-free bread into a loaf and wrap the loaf with aluminum foil. Transfer the foil-wrapped loaf into the preheated oven.

2. Chop the onion.

3. Add the onion and the oil to the stockpot. Stir to combine. Cook on medium low heat, stirring occasionally, until the onion is soft.

4. Add the rosemary, thyme, sage, salt, black pepper, red pepper flakes, and garlic to the stockpot. Stir to combine.

5. Dice the ham into 1/2-inch cubes and add it to the stockpot. Stir to combine.

6. Add the chicken broth (or ham broth) and the bay leaf to the stockpot. Stir to combine. Cover the stockpot with the lid. Increase the heat to medium high until the soup boils then reduce the heat to a gentle simmer.

7. Scrub the carrots under running water, trim their ends, and halve them lengthwise. Slice each half into 3/8-inch thick slices. Add the carrots to the stockpot. Stir to combine.

8. Wash and trim the ends of the celery. Halve each celery rib lengthwise. Slice each half into 3/8-inch thick slices. Add the celery to the stockpot. Stir to combine.

9. Rinse the beans in the colander and allow them to drain thoroughly. Add the beans to the stockpot. Stir gently to combine. Cover the stockpot with the lid and simmer, covered, until the carrots pierce easily with the tines of a fork.

10. While the soup is simmering grate the Parmesan cheese. Transfer the Parmesan cheese to the small serving bowl.

11. When the carrots are tender remove the bay leaf. Serve the soup hot with the (optional) warm gluten-free bread. At serving time, top the soup with a spoonful of grated Parmesan cheese.

Spicy Sausage and Kale Soup

Spicy Italian sausage and hot red pepper flakes give this easy tomato-based soup a flavor kick. Kale and white beans add texture and nutrition. If fresh kale is unavailable you can substitute frozen spinach. This recipe makes a large pot of soup so you'll have enough for lunch the next day.

Ingredients

2 TBSP olive oil or vegetable oil
12 to 16 oz hot Italian sausage in links *
2 cups onion, chopped
 (about 1 large onion)
1/2 tsp salt
1/4 tsp black pepper
1/4 tsp hot red pepper flakes
1 tsp oregano, dried
1/2 tsp granulated garlic *
1 quart gluten-free chicken broth *
1 lb carrots, cut into 1" lengths
1 large bunch kale, washed,
 ribs and stems removed,
 torn in large pieces
 (substitute 8 to 10 oz of pre-washed
 bagged kale or 10 to 12 oz frozen
 spinach)
1 28-oz can tomatoes, crushed or diced,
 (do not drain)
1 15-oz can white beans (Cannellini,
 Great Northern, Navy, or other white
 beans), rinsed and drained

* See **Tips** section

Instructions

1. Add the oil to the stockpot.

2. Add the sausages to the stockpot. Pierce each sausage several times with the tines of a fork to release juices while cooking. Cover the stockpot with the lid. Cook the sausages on medium low heat until they are fully cooked (no pink color when sliced open). Turn once during cooking to brown both sides of the sausages.

3. While the sausages are cooking chop the onion.

4. When the sausages are fully cooked transfer them to a cutting board.

5. Add the onion to the stockpot. Stir to coat the onion with the sausage juices. Increase the heat to medium and cook, stirring occasionally, until the onion is soft.

6. While the onion is cooking slice the sausages into 3/8-inch thick rounds. When the onion is soft add the sliced sausage rounds to the stockpot. Stir to combine.

7. Add the salt, pepper, red pepper flakes, oregano, and the garlic to the stockpot. Stir to coat the onion and sausages with the seasonings.

8. Add the chicken broth to the stockpot. Stir to combine. Cover the stockpot with the lid. Increase the heat to medium high until the soup boils then reduce the heat to a gentle simmer.

9. While the soup is heating scrub the carrots under running water. Trim the ends of the carrots and cut them into 1-inch lengths. Add the carrots to the stockpot. Stir to combine.

Continued

Spicy Sausage and Kale Soup
- Continued -

Cookware and Utensils

6-quart stockpot with lid
Cutting board
Colander

Instructions - continued

10. When the soup is gently simmering rinse the kale in the colander and allow it to drain thoroughly. Remove the stems and tough inner ribs from the kale. Coarsely chop the kale. You may substitute pre-washed bagged kale or frozen spinach. Set aside the kale until the carrots are tender.

11. When the carrots pierce easily with the tines of a fork add the kale to the stockpot. Spoon hot soup over the kale until the kale softens and can be stirred into the soup. Stir to combine.

12. When the kale is completely wilted add the tomatoes (do not drain) to the stockpot. Stir to combine.

13. Rinse the beans in the colander and allow them to drain thoroughly. Add the beans to the stockpot. Stir to combine.

14. Simmer the soup for 15 minutes to combine flavors. Serve the soup hot.

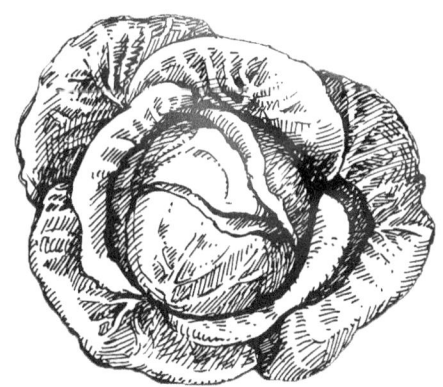

Fall Dinner Ham and Potato Soup

This ham and vegetable soup is ideal for an early autumn dinner when ham, potatoes, and carrots are plentiful. The recipe uses packaged chicken broth for convenience but you can make homemade ham broth quite easily. Simmer a meaty ham bone in a few quarts of water for an hour or two and then strain the broth through a mesh sieve. Unused broth may be stored in the freezer for up to one month.

Ingredients

2 cups onion, chopped
  (about 1 large onion)
2 TBSP vegetable oil
1 tsp salt
1/2 tsp black pepper
1 tsp rosemary, dried
1/2 tsp thyme, dried
1/2 tsp marjoram, dried
1 1/2 tsp granulated garlic *
3 carrots, ends trimmed,
  cut into 1" lengths
1 1/2 lbs potatoes, cut into 1" cubes
16 oz ham, diced into 3/4" cubes *
1 quart gluten-free chicken broth
  or ham broth *
1 bay leaf

* See *Tips* section

Cookware and Utensils

6-quart stockpot with lid
Small bowl

Instructions

1. Chop the onion.

2. Add the onion and the oil to the stockpot. Stir to combine. Cook on medium heat, stirring occasionally, until the onion is soft.

3. While the onion is cooking add the salt, pepper, rosemary, thyme, marjoram, and garlic to the small bowl. Stir to combine.

4. Scrub the carrots under running water and trim their ends. Cut the carrots into 1-inch lengths. When the onion is soft add the carrots to the stockpot. Stir to combine.

5. Scrub the potatoes under running water. Cut the potatoes into 1-inch cubes. Add the potatoes to the stockpot. Stir to combine.

6. Dice the ham into 3/4-inch cubes. Add the ham to the stockpot. Stir to combine.

7. Add the mixed seasonings to the stockpot. Stir to coat the ham and vegetable mixture with the seasonings.

8. Add the chicken broth (or ham broth) and the bay leaf to the stockpot. Stir to combine. Cover the stockpot with the lid. Increase the heat to medium high until the soup boils then reduce the heat to a gentle simmer.

9. Simmer the soup, covered, until the vegetables pierce easily with the tines of a fork.

10. When the vegetables are tender remove the bay leaf. Serve the soup hot.

Easy French Cassoulet

Cassoulet (CASS-sue-lay) is the French equivalent of 'pork and beans'. It is a traditional casserole that originated in the south of France. A simple but time-consuming peasant dish, cassoulet consists of white beans slow-cooked with pork, goose, or duck meat. This quick and easy version uses mild-flavored sausages and lots of herbs and garlic for a savory, filling dish.

Ingredients

4 slices bacon, cut into 1/2" pieces
1 lb mild-flavored sausage in casings *
  (mild Italian, chicken Parmesan,
  or other mild-flavored sausage)
1 cup onion chopped
  (about 1/2 of a large onion)
4 cloves garlic, chopped
2 TBSP olive oil or vegetable oil
1/2 tsp thyme, dried
1/2 tsp rosemary, dried
1/2 tsp salt
1/4 tsp black pepper
2 cups gluten-free chicken broth *
3 15-oz cans white beans (Cannellini,
  Great Northern, Navy, or other
  white beans), rinsed and drained

* See *Tips* section

Cookware and Utensils

6-quart stockpot with lid
Cutting board
Colander

Instructions

1. Cut the bacon into 1/2-inch pieces. Add the bacon to the stockpot. Crisp the bacon on medium heat, stirring frequently.

2. When the bacon is crisp move it to one side of the stockpot. Add the sausages to the stockpot. Pierce each sausage several times with the tines of a fork to release juices while cooking. Cover the stockpot with the lid. Reduce the heat to medium low and cook the sausages until they are fully cooked (no pink color when sliced open). Turn once during cooking to brown both sides of the sausages.

3. While the sausages are cooking chop the onion and the garlic.

4. When the sausages are fully cooked transfer them to a cutting board.

5. Add the oil, onion, garlic, thyme, rosemary, salt, and pepper to the stockpot. Stir to combine. Cover the stockpot with the lid. Cook on medium low heat until the onion is soft. Stir occasionally.

6. While the onion is cooking slice the sausages into 3/8-inch thick rounds. When the onion is soft add the sliced sausage rounds to the stockpot. Stir to combine.

7. Add the chicken broth to the stockpot. Stir to combine.

8. Drain and rinse the beans in a colander. Allow the beans to drain thoroughly then add the beans to the stockpot. Stir gently to combine.

9. Increase the heat to medium high. Bring the mixture to a boil then reduce the heat to a gentle simmer. Simmer the cassoulet, uncovered, for 10 minutes to combine flavors and reduce the broth. Serve the cassoulet hot.

Hearty Minestrone Soup in a Flash

Minestrone is an Italian vegetable soup whose recipe is so old that it predates the Roman Empire. An example of 'Cucina Povera' or 'poor kitchen' cuisine, this humble peasant soup began as a pot of vegetables served with a porridge. As the Italians prospered they added meats to the soup. With the opening of trade routes to the New World new foods such as tomatoes and potatoes found their way into the cooking pot.

Ingredients

10 to 12 oz frozen mixed vegetables
6 slices bacon (about 8 oz by weight)
1 cup onion, chopped
 (about 1/2 of a large onion)
1 lb potatoes, cut into 1/2" cubes
1 tsp oregano, dried
1/2 tsp basil, dried
1/2 tsp thyme, dried
1 tsp Italian seasoning
1 1/2 tsp granulated garlic *
1 tsp salt
1/2 tsp black pepper
1/4 tsp hot red pepper flakes
1 28-oz can tomatoes, diced or crushed
 (do not drain)
2 cups water
1 bay leaf
1 15-oz can white beans (Navy,
 Great Northern, Cannellini
 or other white beans),
 rinsed and drained
1/4 cup grated Parmesan cheese *

* See **Tips** section

For the Optional Garlic Toast

8 slices gluten-free bread
2 TBSP olive oil
2 tsp granulated garlic *

Instructions

1. If you will be making the (optional) garlic toast then preheat the oven to 300 degrees F.

2. Transfer the frozen mixed vegetables to the countertop to thaw while you are making the soup.

3. Cut the bacon into 1/2-inch pieces. Add the bacon to the stockpot. Crisp the bacon on medium heat, stirring frequently.

4. While the bacon is crisping chop the onion. When the bacon is crisp add the onion to the stockpot. Stir to combine. Lower the heat to medium low and continue cooking, stirring occasionally, until the onion is soft.

5. Peel the potatoes if desired. Cut the potatoes into 1/2-inch cubes and add them to the stockpot. Stir to combine.

6. Add the oregano, basil, thyme, Italian seasoning, garlic, salt, pepper, and red pepper flakes to a small bowl. Stir to combine.

7. Add the mixed seasonings to the stockpot. Stir to coat the vegetables with the seasonings.

8. Add the tomatoes (do not drain), 2 cups of water, and the frozen mixed vegetables to the stockpot. Stir to combine.

9. Add the bay leaf to the stockpot and submerge it below the surface of the liquid. Cover the stockpot with the lid. Increase the heat to medium high until the soup boils then reduce the heat to a gentle simmer.

10. Rinse and drain the beans in the colander. Add the beans to the stockpot. Stir gently to combine. Cover the stockpot with the lid and simmer for 20 minutes to combine flavors.

Continued

Hearty Minestrone Soup in a Flash
- Continued -

This hearty version of this ancient rustic soup stays true to the original's roots by loading up on vegetables and flavoring the soup with savory bacon.

Cookware and Utensils

6-qt stockpot with lid
Vegetable peeler or paring knife
  (optional)
Small bowl for seasonings
Colander
Metal baking sheet (optional)
Aluminum foil or parchment paper
  (optional)
Small bowl for olive oil (optional)
Basting brush (optional)
Shredder/grater
  (if not using pre-grated cheese)
Small serving bowl

Instructions - continued

11. If you are making the optional garlic toast then line a baking sheet with aluminum foil or parchment paper. Arrange the gluten-free bread in a single layer on the lined baking sheet.

12. Transfer the baking sheet to the oven. Toast the first side of the bread until slightly crunchy (about 10 minutes).

13. Remove the baking sheet from the oven. Flip each slice of bread. Baste the top sides of the bread slices with 2 tablespoons of olive oil. Sprinkle the bread slices lightly with 2 teaspoons of granulated garlic. Return the baking sheet to the oven. Toast the bread until the top side of the bread is light golden brown (about 10 minutes). Turn off the oven and keep the toast warm in the oven until serving time.

14. Grate the Parmesan cheese if necessary and transfer it to a small serving bowl.

15. After the soup has simmered for 20 minutes check the potatoes for doneness. The potatoes are done when they pierce easily with the tines of a fork.

16. When the potatoes are tender remove the bay leaf. Serve the soup hot with (optional) warm garlic bread and a spoonful of Parmesan cheese sprinkled over the top.

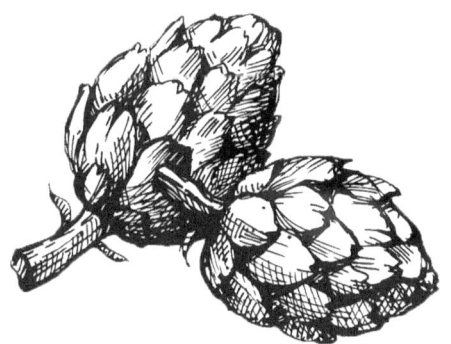

Best Ever Pizza Soup

Sometimes you crave the taste of pizza without the fuss. This easy soup has all the flavors of a sausage, pepperoni, and mushroom pizza without the hassle of making a gluten-free crust. If you like green bell pepper on your pizza then feel free to add it along with any other favorite pizza toppings like sliced black olives, red onion sliced into crescents, red bell pepper, banana peppers, diced ham, Canadian bacon, canned artichoke, or sliced pepperoncini peppers.

Ingredients

12 to 16 oz mild Italian sausage *
6 oz pepperoni, thinly sliced,
　slices cut in half *
1/2 cup onion, finely chopped
4 cloves garlic, finely chopped
1 green bell pepper, washed and seeded,
　diced into 1/2" pieces (optional)
8 oz white button mushrooms,
　washed and thinly sliced
3/4 tsp salt
1 tsp Italian seasoning
1 tsp oregano, dried
1/2 tsp basil, dried
1/4 tsp hot red pepper flakes
1/4 tsp fennel seed, slightly crushed
　(optional)
1 28-oz can tomatoes, diced or crushed
　(do not drain)
1 15-oz can tomato sauce
　(substitute two 8-oz cans tomato sauce)
2 cups water
3 TBSP grated Parmesan cheese *
1 cup shredded Mozzarella cheese
　(about 4 oz by weight) *

* See *Tips* section

Instructions

1. Remove the sausage from its casings if necessary. Add the sausage to the stockpot, breaking it into small chunks, about 3/4-inch in size. Brown the sausage on medium heat, stirring occasionally.

2. While the sausage is browning slice the pepperoni into thin slices (skip this step if you have purchased pre-sliced pepperoni).

3. Cut the pepperoni slices in half.

4. Finely chop the onion and garlic.

5. If you will be adding the (optional) bell pepper then wash, seed, and dice it into 1/2-inch pieces. Prepare any other optional ingredients by chopping them into bite-size pieces.

6. Rinse the mushrooms in the colander and allow them to drain thoroughly. Slice the mushrooms thinly.

7. When the sausage is cooked all the way through (no pink color) drain some of the grease from the stockpot by moving the stockpot to a cool unused burner, tipping it away from you to pool the grease, then carefully spooning the grease into a small heatproof bowl. Reserve about a tablespoon of sausage drippings in the stockpot. Allow the unused grease to cool before disposing.

8. Return the stockpot to the heated burner. Add the pepperoni, onion, garlic, bell pepper (optional), and any other additional pizza topping ingredients you desire to the stockpot. Stir to combine. Cook on medium heat, stirring occasionally, until the onion begins to soften.

9. When the onion begins to soften add the mushrooms to the stockpot. Stir to combine. Cover the stockpot with the lid. Cook, covered, on medium heat until the mushrooms are soft. Stir occasionally.

Continued

Best Ever Pizza Soup
- Continued -

Cookware and Utensils

6-quart stockpot with lid
Colander
Small heatproof bowl
Mortar and pestle or small ceramic bowl
  (if adding the optional crushed
  fennel seed)
Shredder/grater
  (if not using pre-grated or
  pre-shredded cheese)

Instructions - continued

10. When the mushrooms are soft add the salt, Italian seasoning, oregano, basil, and red pepper flakes to the stockpot. Stir to combine.

11. If you will be adding the optional fennel seeds then lightly crush them with a mortar and pestle before adding them to the stockpot. If you don't have a mortar and pestle use the back side of a table spoon to crush the fennel seeds against the inside of a small ceramic bowl. You don't need to break apart the seeds into smaller pieces, just apply enough pressure to crack the tough seed coating. Lightly crushing the seeds allows their flavor to disperse more quickly into the soup.

12. Add the canned tomatoes (do not drain), the tomato sauce, and 2 cups of water to the stockpot. Stir to combine. Cover the stockpot with the lid. Increase the heat to medium high until the soup boils then reduce the heat to a gentle simmer. Simmer the soup for 15 minutes to combine flavors. Stir occasionally.

13. While the soup is simmering grate the Parmesan cheese and shred the Mozzarella cheese (if not using pre-grated or pre-shredded cheese).

14. After the soup is done simmering add the Parmesan cheese to the stockpot. Stir to combine.

15. Serve the soup hot. Ladle the soup into serving bowls and top each bowl with a handful of shredded Mozzarella cheese.

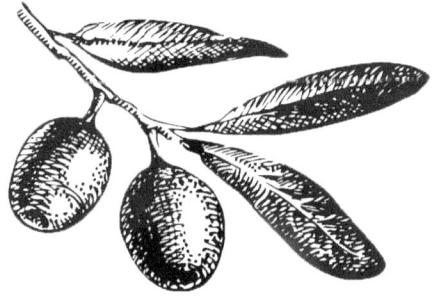

Pork

Tuscan Sausage and Bean Soup

This quick and easy sausage and white bean soup gets its origins from rustic soups that were served in the Tuscany region of Italy. Choose a mild (sweet) Italian sausage for this recipe. Add the optional fennel seed for extra flavor.

Ingredients

1 TBSP olive oil or vegetable oil
1 lb mild Italian sausage, in links *
2 cups onion, chopped
   (about 1 large onion)
2 carrots, trimmed and halved
   lengthwise, each half sliced
   into 3/8" thick slices
1 1/4 tsp salt
1/4 tsp black pepper
1 tsp Italian seasoning
1/2 tsp rosemary, dried
1 1/2 tsp granulated garlic *
1/4 tsp hot red pepper flakes
1/4 tsp fennel seed, slightly crushed
   (optional)
1 quart gluten-free chicken broth *
1 bay leaf
2 15-oz cans white beans (Cannellini,
   Great Northern, Navy, or other white
   beans), rinsed and drained
1/4 cup grated Parmesan cheese *

* See **Tips** section

Instructions

1. Add the oil to the stockpot.

2. Arrange the sausages in a single layer on the bottom of the stockpot. Pierce each sausage several times with the tines of a fork to release juices while cooking. Cover the stockpot with the lid. Cook the sausages on medium low heat, turning once during cooking to brown both sides of the sausages.

3. While the sausages are cooking chop the onion.

4. Scrub the carrots under running water, trim their ends, and slice them in half lengthwise. Slice each half into 3/8-inch thick slices.

5. When the sausages are fully cooked (no pink color when sliced open) transfer them to a cutting board to cool. Drain some of the grease from the stockpot by moving the stockpot to a cool unused burner, tipping it away from you to pool the grease, then carefully spooning the grease into a small heatproof bowl. Reserve about a tablespoon of sausage drippings in the stockpot. Allow the unused grease to cool before disposing.

6. Return the stockpot to the heated burner. Add the onion and the carrots to the stockpot. Stir to combine. Increase the heat to medium and cook, stirring occasionally, until the onion is soft.

7. While the onion is cooking slice the sausages into 3/8-inch thick rounds.

8. When the onion is soft add the salt, pepper, Italian seasoning, rosemary, garlic, and red pepper flakes to the stockpot. Stir to combine.

Continued

Tuscan Sausage and Bean Soup
- Continued -

Cookware and Utensils

6-quart stockpot with lid
Cutting board
Small heatproof bowl
Mortar and pestle or small ceramic bowl
  (if adding the optional crushed
  fennel seed)
Colander
Shredder/grater
  (if not using pre-grated cheese)
Small serving bowl

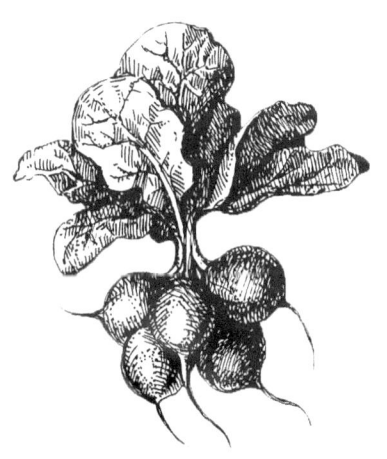

Instructions - continued

9. If you will be adding the optional fennel seeds then lightly crush them with a mortar and pestle before adding them to the stockpot. If you don't have a mortar and pestle use the back side of a table spoon to crush the fennel seeds against the inside of a small ceramic bowl. You don't need to break apart the seeds into smaller pieces, just apply enough pressure to crack the tough seed coating. Lightly crushing the seeds allows their flavor to disperse more quickly into the soup.

10. Add the sliced sausages to the stockpot. Stir to combine.

11. Add the chicken broth and the bay leaf to the stockpot. Stir to combine. Cover the stockpot with the lid. Increase the heat to medium high until the soup boils then reduce the heat to a gentle simmer. Stir occasionally.

12. Rinse the beans in the colander and allow them to drain thoroughly. When the beans are well drained add them to the stockpot. Stir to combine. Continue simmering the soup until the carrots pierce easily with the tines of a fork.

13. While the soup is simmering grate the Parmesan cheese if necessary and transfer it to the small serving bowl.

14. When the carrots are tender remove the bay leaf. Serve the soup hot with a spoonful of Parmesan cheese sprinkled over the top.

Minnesota Wild Rice Soup

Wild rice is not a true rice but the seeds of a grass that grows in the shallow fresh water lakes and slow-flowing streams of Minnesota. It was traditionally harvested by Native American Indians who used long wooden sticks to knock the ripe seeds off the tall grass into the bottom of canoes. This cream-based soup is inspired by the Wild Rice Soup served at Minnesota's Lake Itasca Douglas Lodge where the headwaters of the Mississippi River are located.

Ingredients

6 oz wild rice, uncooked
  (about 3/4 cup)
3 cups water
6 slices bacon, cut into 1/2" pieces
1 1/4 cups onion, finely chopped
8 oz white button mushrooms,
  washed and sliced
2 ribs celery, sliced thinly into 3/8" slices
3 carrots, halved lengthwise,
  sliced into 3/8" slices
3/4 tsp thyme, dried
1/4 tsp marjoram, dried
1 3/4 tsp salt
1/2 tsp black pepper
1 tsp granulated garlic *
2 cups gluten-free chicken broth *
1/4 cup white wine (substitute water)
1 cup mashed potato flakes
2 cups half-and-half

* See *Tips* section

Instructions

1. Rinse the wild rice in the colander or mesh sieve and drain well.

2. Add the drained wild rice and 3 cups of water to the 2-quart saucepan. Cover the saucepan with the lid. Heat on high heat until the water boils then reduce the heat to a gentle simmer. Simmer the rice, covered, until the grains begin to burst and the rice tastes chewy but is not yet mushy (about 40 minutes).

3. While the rice is cooking cut the bacon into 1/2-inch pieces. Add the bacon to the stockpot. Crisp the bacon on medium heat, stirring frequently.

4. Finely chop the onion.

5. Rinse the mushrooms in the colander or mesh sieve and allow them to drain thoroughly. Slice the mushrooms.

6. Wash the celery ribs and trim their ends. Slice the celery into 3/8-inch thick slices.

7. Scrub the carrots under running water and trim their ends. Cut the carrots in half lengthwise. Slice each half into 3/8-inch thick slices.

8. When the bacon is crisp turn off the heat. Drain some of the grease from the stockpot by moving the stockpot to a cool unused burner, tipping the stockpot away from you to pool the grease, then carefully spooning the grease into a small heatproof bowl. Reserve about two tablespoons of bacon drippings in the stockpot. Allow the unused grease to cool before disposing.

9. Return the stockpot to the heated burner. Add the onion and the mushrooms to the stockpot. Stir to coat the onion and mushrooms with the bacon drippings. Cook on medium heat, stirring occasionally, until the onion is soft.

10. When the onion is soft add the thyme, marjoram, salt, pepper, and garlic to the stockpot. Stir to combine.

Continued

Minnesota Wild Rice Soup
- Continued -

Our recipe combines this Native American food with mushrooms and bacon for a hearty, flavorful soup. If you don't own a 2-quart saucepan you can cook the wild rice in the stockpot first. Drain the wild rice in the colander then proceed with the recipe.

Cookware and Utensils

Metal heat-proof colander
  or large mesh sieve
2-quart saucepan with lid
6-quart stockpot with lid
Small heatproof bowl

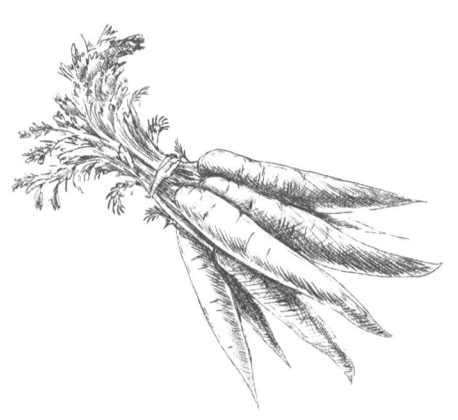

Instructions

11. Add the chicken broth to the stockpot. Stir to combine.

12. Add the celery and the carrots to the stockpot. Stir to combine. Cover the stockpot with the lid. Increase the heat to medium high until the broth begins to boil then reduce the heat to a gentle simmer. Simmer, covered, until the carrots pierce easily with the tines of a fork.

13. When the carrots are tender turn off the heat to the stockpot. Cover the stockpot with the lid.

14. After the wild rice has simmered for 40 minutes test it for doneness. The wild rice is done when the grains have split open and are chewy to the taste but not hard or mushy. Not all of the water will be absorbed. When the wild rice is done remove the saucepan from the stove and drain the wild rice in a heatproof metal colander or metal mesh sieve. Set aside the drained wild rice.

15. Add the white wine (substitute water) to the stockpot. Stir to combine.

16. Sprinkle the mashed potato flakes over the stockpot. Let them rehydrate for a minute or two then stir to combine. Wait another minute then stir again to completely dissolve the mashed potato flakes into the soup.

17. Add the drained wild rice to the stockpot. Stir to combine.

18. Add the half-and-half to the stockpot. Stir to combine. Heat the soup on medium low heat until it is at serving temperature. Do not boil the soup or the cream will separate. Serve hot.

Spicy Chorizo Corn Chowder

This mildly-spiced chowder gets its kick from Mexican chorizo sausage, an uncooked spicy sausage that differs from Spanish chorizo which is a smoked dried sausage. Green chilis, savory red onion, and tangy lime give this chowder lots of flavor while corn and diced potato make it a filling one-pot meal. If you can't find Mexican chorizo you can substitute one pound of readily-available hot Italian sausage, some cayenne pepper, and additional granulated garlic.

Ingredients

12 to 16 oz Mexican chorizo sausage, casings removed *
(substitute 1 lb hot Italian sausage *
 + 1/4 tsp cayenne pepper
 + 1 tsp granulated garlic *)
1 cup red onion, sliced into crescents
1 red bell pepper, seeded and cut into 1/2" strips, strips halved
2 large potatoes, peeled and cut into 1" cubes
1 4-oz can diced mild green chilis (do not drain)
1 tsp oregano, dried (use Mexican oregano if available)
1/2 tsp basil, dried
1/2 tsp granulated garlic *
1 tsp salt
1 tsp ground cumin
3 cups gluten-free chicken broth *
1 lime, juiced (about 1 TBSP juice)
3/4 cup mashed potato flakes
2 cups frozen corn kernels
1 1/2 cups half-and-half

* See **Tips** section

Cookware and Utensils

6-quart stockpot with lid
Vegetable peeler or paring knife
Citrus juicer

Instructions

1. Remove the chorizo (or hot Italian sausage) from its casings if necessary and break it into small pieces, about 3/4-inch in size. Add the chorizo to the stockpot. Brown the chorizo on medium heat. Stir occasionally.

2. While the chorizo is cooking slice the red onion into thin crescents. Add the red onion to the stockpot. Stir to combine.

3. Wash, seed, and cut the bell pepper into 1/2-inch thick strips. Cut each strip in half. Add the bell pepper to the stockpot. Stir to combine.

4. Peel the potatoes and cut them into 1-inch cubes. Set aside the potatoes.

5. After the chorizo is fully cooked (no pink color) add the canned chilis to the stockpot (do not drain). Stir to combine.

6. Add the oregano, basil, garlic, salt, and cumin to the stockpot. Stir to coat the sausage and vegetables with the seasonings.

7. If you are substituting hot Italian sausage for chorizo then add the 1/4 teaspoon of cayenne pepper and the extra teaspoon of granulated garlic at this time. Stir to combine.

8. Add the chicken broth and the potatoes to the stockpot. Stir to combine. Cover the stockpot with the lid. Increase the heat to medium high until the mixture boils then reduce the heat to a gentle simmer. Simmer, stirring occasionally, until the potatoes are tender when pierced with the tines of a fork.

9. While the chowder is simmering juice the lime.

10. When the potatoes pierce easily with the tines of a fork add the mashed potato flakes to the stockpot. Stir to combine.

11. Add the lime juice and the corn kernels to the stockpot. Stir to combine.

12. Add the half-and-half to the stockpot. Stir to combine. Reduce the heat to medium low. Cover the stockpot with the lid and gently heat the chowder to serving temperature. Stir occasionally. Do not boil the chowder or the cream will separate. Serve the chowder hot.

Seafood

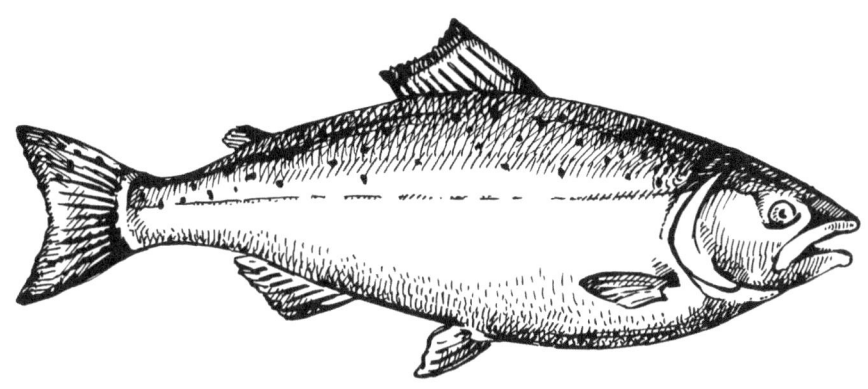

Meals in a Skillet

154   *Cheesy Salmon Skillet*
155   *Tasty Tuna Macaroni Skillet*
156   *Tuna Mushroom Skillet*

Soups and Stews

157   *New England Clam Chowder*
158   *Herbed Salmon Chowder*
160   *Manhattan Clam Chowder*
161   *Chipotle Shrimp and Avocado Soup*
162   *Easy Cioppino*
164   *Thai Shrimp and Noodle Soup*
166   *Shrimp and Rice Gumbo*

Cheesy Salmon Skillet

Salmon is 'the other canned fish' and is frequently overlooked which is a shame because not only does it taste great but it is also good for you. Salmon is high in protein, Omega-3 fatty acids, vitamin D, and B vitamins. Use a good quality canned salmon as it is the star of the show in this skillet.

Ingredients

3 TBSP butter
1/4 cup onion, finely chopped
1 cup water, heated
1 tsp salt
1/2 tsp thyme, dried
1/2 tsp granulated garlic *
10 to 12 oz skinless, boneless canned
  salmon, packed in water *
1 3/4 cups milk *
8 oz gluten-free pasta **
2 cups shredded Monterey Jack cheese *
  (about 8 oz measured by weight)
1 1/2 cups frozen cut green beans

* See *Tips* section
** See *Measuring Pasta* section

Cookware and Utensils

12-inch skillet with lid
Microwave-safe liquid measuring cup
  (1-cup size or larger)
Small bowl
Shredder/grater
  (if not using pre-shredded cheese)

Instructions

1. Add the butter to the skillet. Melt the butter on low heat.

2. Finely chop the onion and add it to the melted butter. Cook on medium heat, stirring frequently, until the onion is soft.

3. While the onion is cooking microwave 1 cup of water on high power for 1 minute.

4. When the onion is soft add the salt, thyme, and garlic to the onion. Stir to combine.

5. Drain the broth from the canned salmon into the small bowl. Add 3 tablespoons of the salmon broth to the onion mixture. Stir to combine. Discard unused salmon broth.

6. Add the hot water and the milk to the onion mixture. Stir to combine.

7. Add the gluten-free pasta to the skillet. Stir to combine. Cover the skillet with the lid. Increase the heat to medium high until the mixture boils then reduce the heat to a gentle simmer.

8. Most gluten-free pastas cook in 7 to 12 minutes. Stir the mixture frequently, checking every 3 to 4 minutes until the pasta is cooked to your taste.

9. While the pasta is cooking shred the Monterey Jack cheese (if not using pre-shredded cheese).

10. When the pasta is cooked to the desired doneness stir in the green beans. Cover the skillet with the lid. Heat for a few minutes until the green beans are tender crisp.

11. Add the shredded cheese to the skillet. Stir to combine. Cover the skillet with the lid. Turn off the heat and allow the cheese to fully melt. Stir again to mix the cheese evenly.

12. Break the drained salmon into large chunks. Discard any pieces of skin or fish bones. Gently fold the salmon chunks into the mixture until they are evenly distributed, using care to keep the salmon from breaking up too much. Serve immediately.

Tasty Tuna Macaroni Skillet

This luscious skillet is loaded with tuna and gets its creaminess from real Parmesan cheese. For the best flavor use real butter instead of margarine.

Ingredients

1/2 cup onion, chopped
  (about 1/4 of a large onion)
2 TBSP butter
1 cup water, heated
1 tsp salt
1/4 tsp black pepper
2 tsp dried parsley flakes
2 cups milk *
8 oz gluten-free pasta **
10 to 12 oz tuna, packed in water *
3/4 cup grated Parmesan cheese *
1 cup frozen peas and carrots

* See **Tips** section
** See **Measuring Pasta** section

Cookware and Utensils

12-inch skillet with lid
Microwave-safe liquid measuring cup
  (1-cup size or larger)
Colander
Shredder/grater
  (if not using pre-grated cheese)

Instructions

1. Chop the onion.

2. Add the butter and the onion to the skillet. Cook on low heat until the onion is soft. Stir frequently.

3. While the onion is cooking microwave 1 cup of water on high power for 1 minute.

4. When the onion is soft add the salt, pepper, and parsley flakes to the skillet. Stir to combine.

5. Add the hot water and the milk to the skillet. Stir to combine.

6. Add the gluten-free pasta to the skillet. Stir to combine. Cover the skillet with the lid. Increase the heat to medium high until the mixture boils then reduce the heat to a gentle simmer.

7. Most gluten-free pastas cook in 7 to 12 minutes. Stir the mixture frequently, checking every 3 to 4 minutes until the pasta is cooked to your taste.

8. While the pasta is cooking drain the water from the tuna.

9. Grate the Parmesan cheese (if not using pre-grated cheese).

10. When the pasta is cooked to the desired doneness stir in the frozen peas and carrots. Cover the skillet with the lid and heat for a few minutes until the vegetables are tender crisp.

11. Stir in the grated Parmesan cheese. Cover the skillet with the lid. Reduce the heat to low and heat for a few minutes to melt the cheese. Stir to combine the melted cheese.

12. Break the drained tuna into large chunks. Gently fold the tuna chunks into the mixture until they are evenly distributed, using care to keep the tuna from breaking up too much. Serve immediately.

Tuna Mushroom Skillet

When you went gluten-free the option to 'open a can of cream of mushroom soup' became limited making it harder to prepare many traditional casserole recipes. This creamy tuna and mushroom casserole-in-a-skillet is healthier for you and has more flavor than those casseroles made with bland prepared cream soups. It uses half a pound of fresh mushrooms and tuna packed in water to keep the calories low and the flavor high.

Ingredients

1 cup onion, chopped
  (about 1/2 of a large onion)
3 TBSP butter
8 oz white button mushrooms,
  washed and sliced
1 cup water, heated
1 tsp salt
1/4 tsp thyme, dried
1/4 tsp black pepper
1/2 tsp marjoram, dried
1/2 tsp granulated garlic *
2 cups milk *
8 oz gluten-free pasta **
10 to 12 oz tuna, packed in water *
2 cups shredded Monterey Jack cheese *
  (about 8 oz measured by weight)
1 1/2 cups frozen cut green beans

* See *Tips* section
** See *Measuring Pasta* section

Cookware and Utensils

12-inch skillet with lid
Colander
Microwave-safe liquid measuring cup
  (1-cup size or larger)
Shredder/grater
  (if not using pre-shredded cheese)

Instructions

1. Chop the onion.

2. Add the butter and the onion to the skillet. Cook on low heat until the onion is soft. Stir frequently.

3. Rinse the mushrooms and allow them to drain. Slice the mushrooms. Add the sliced mushrooms to the skillet. Stir to combine. Cover the skillet with the lid. Increase the heat to medium and continue cooking until the mushrooms are soft. Stir occasionally.

4. While the onion and mushroom mixture is cooking microwave 1 cup of water on high power for 1 minute.

5. When the mushrooms are soft add the salt, thyme, pepper, marjoram, and garlic to the mushroom and onion mixture. Stir to coat the mushrooms and onions with the seasonings.

6. Add the hot water and the milk to the mushroom and onion mixture. Stir to combine.

7. Add the gluten-free pasta to the skillet. Stir to combine. Cover the skillet with the lid. Increase the heat to medium high until the mixture boils then reduce the heat to a gentle simmer.

8. Most gluten-free pastas cook in 7 to 12 minutes. Stir the mixture frequently, checking every 3 to 4 minutes until the pasta is cooked to your taste.

9. While the pasta is cooking drain the water from the tuna.

10. Shred the Monterey Jack cheese (if not using pre-shredded cheese).

11. When the pasta is cooked to the desired doneness stir in the green beans. Cover the skillet with the lid and heat for a few minutes until the beans are tender crisp.

12. Stir in the shredded Monterey Jack cheese. Cover the skillet with the lid. Turn off the heat and allow the cheese to fully melt. Stir to combine.

13. Break the drained tuna into large chunks. Gently fold the tuna chunks into the mixture until they are evenly distributed, using care to keep the tuna from breaking up too much. Serve immediately.

New England Clam Chowder

When it comes to Clam Chowder folks have strong preferences. The 'New England' version of this clam soup is milk-based. The 'Manhattan' version features a spicy tomato base. The debate over which was best was so contentious that in 1939 a bill was introduced into the Maine state legislature attempting to make it illegal to add tomatoes to 'Clam Chowder'. This recipe is the version favored by the folks in Maine.

Ingredients

4 strips bacon, cut into 1/2" pieces
1/2 cup onion, chopped
2 ribs celery,
　sliced thinly into 3/8" thick slices
3 carrots, trimmed and halved
　lengthwise, halves sliced
　into 3/8" thick slices
1 1/2 lbs potatoes, peeled and cut
　into 1/2" cubes
1 10-oz can baby clams
　(reserve 1/2 cup clam broth)
1/2 tsp thyme, dried
1 1/2 tsp salt
1/4 tsp black pepper
1 8-oz bottle clam juice *
2 cups gluten-free chicken broth *
1 bay leaf
2 TBSP butter
1/2 cup white wine (substitute water)
1 1/2 cups mashed potato flakes
1 1/2 cups half-and-half

* See *Tips* section

Cookware and Utensils

6-quart stockpot with lid
Vegetable peeler or paring knife
Mesh sieve
Liquid measuring cup,
　(1-cup size or larger)

Instructions

1. Cut the bacon into 1/2-inch pieces and add it to the stockpot. Crisp the bacon on medium heat. Stir frequently.

2. While the bacon is crisping chop the onion. Trim the ends of the celery and slice it into 3/8-inch thick slices. Scrub the carrots under running water. Halve the carrots lengthwise then slice each half into 3/8-inch thick slices. Peel the potatoes if desired and cut them into 1/2-inch cubes.

3. When the bacon is crisp add the onion, celery, carrots, and potatoes to the stockpot. Stir to combine. Cook on medium heat, stirring occasionally, until the onion is soft.

4. While the vegetables are cooking drain the clams in a mesh sieve positioned over a liquid measuring cup to reserve the clam broth. Set aside the clam broth. Rinse the clams and allow them to drain thoroughly. Inspect the clams for shell fragments or foreign matter and remove if necessary.

5. When the onion is soft add the thyme, salt, pepper, bottled clam juice, 1/2 cup of the reserved clam broth, chicken broth, and the bay leaf to the stockpot. Stir to combine. Submerge the bay leaf in the liquid. Cover the stockpot with the lid. Increase the heat to medium high until the mixture boils then reduce the heat to a gentle simmer. Simmer until the carrots and potatoes pierce easily with the tines of a fork. Stir occasionally.

6. When the carrots and potatoes are tender remove the bay leaf. Add the butter to the stockpot. Stir to combine.

7. Add the white wine (substitute water) and the drained clams to the stockpot. Stir gently to combine.

8. Sprinkle the mashed potato flakes over the stockpot. Stir gently to combine. Allow the mashed potato flakes to rehydrate for a minute or two then stir gently again to break up any remaining flakes.

9. Add the half-and-half to the stockpot. Stir to combine. Reduce the heat to low. Gently heat the chowder to serving temperature. Do not boil or the cream will separate. When the chowder is at serving temperature serve immediately.

Seafood

Herbed Salmon Chowder

America's East Coast is famous for its clam chowders. The West Coast has their own chowder that makes use of the abundant salmon found in the Pacific Northwest's pristine rivers and the cold waters of the northernmost reaches of the Pacific Ocean. This recipe uses canned salmon for convenience but feel free to use fresh salmon if it's available. Just ensure that the salmon is cooked thoroughly before adding the half-and-half. Choose a good quality canned salmon for this recipe.

Ingredients

3 TBSP butter
3/4 cup onion, chopped
2 ribs celery, sliced thinly into 3/8" thick slices
2 carrots, trimmed and halved lengthwise, halves sliced into 3/8" thick slices
1 lb potatoes, peeled and cut into 1/2" cubes
1 1/2 tsp salt
1/4 tsp black pepper
1/2 tsp thyme, dried
2 tsp dried parsley flakes
1/2 tsp granulated garlic *
2 cups gluten-free chicken broth *
1/2 cup white wine (substitute water)
1 bay leaf
3/4 cup mashed potato flakes
1 15-oz can salmon, broth drained and reserved, skin and bones removed (substitute 12 oz fresh salmon fillet, skinned and boned, cut into 1" pieces)
1 cup half-and-half

* See **Tips** section

Instructions

1. Add the butter to the stockpot. Melt the butter on low heat.

2. Chop the onion and add it to the stockpot. Stir to combine. Increase the heat to medium low and cook, stirring occasionally, until the onion is soft.

3. While the onion is cooking wash and trim the ends from the celery. Slice the celery into 3/8-inch thick slices. Add the celery to the stockpot. Stir to combine.

4. Scrub the carrots under running water, trim their ends and halve them lengthwise. Slice each half into 3/8-inch thick slices. Add the carrots to the stockpot. Stir to combine.

5. Scrub the potatoes under running water. Peel the potatoes if desired. Cut the potatoes into 1/2-inch cubes. Add the potatoes to the stockpot. Stir to combine.

6. Add the salt, pepper, thyme, parsley, and garlic to the stockpot. Stir to coat the vegetables with the seasonings.

7. Add the chicken broth, white wine (substitute water), and the bay leaf to the stockpot. Stir to combine. Cover the stockpot with the lid. Increase the heat to medium high until the broth boils then reduce the heat to a gentle simmer. Simmer, covered, until the carrots and potatoes pierce easily with the tines of a fork.

8. When the carrots and potatoes are tender remove the bay leaf. Sprinkle the mashed potato flakes over the stockpot. Let the mashed potato flakes rehydrate for a minute or two then stir until they are completely dissolved into the broth.

9. If using canned salmon skip to the next step. If using fresh salmon then skin, bone, and cut the salmon fillet into 1-inch pieces. Add the salmon pieces to the stockpot. Stir gently to combine.

Continued

Herbed Salmon Chowder
- Continued -

Cookware and Utensils

6-quart stockpot with lid
Vegetable peeler or paring knife (optional)
Mesh sieve
Small bowl
Medium bowl

Instructions - continued

10. If using canned salmon place a mesh sieve over the small bowl. Drain the canned salmon over the mesh sieve, reserving all of the salmon broth. Add the reserved salmon broth to the stockpot. Stir to combine.

11. Transfer the canned salmon to the medium bowl. Remove the skin and bones from the canned salmon and discard. Break the canned salmon into 1-inch chunks. Set aside the canned salmon.

12. Add the half-and-half to the stockpot (if using fresh salmon wait until the salmon is completely cooked before adding the half-and-half). Stir gently to combine.

13. Add the canned salmon chunks to the stockpot. Stir gently to combine. Heat on medium low heat to serving temperature. Do not boil the chowder or the cream will separate.

14. Serve the chowder hot. This chowder is best eaten on the same day it is prepared.

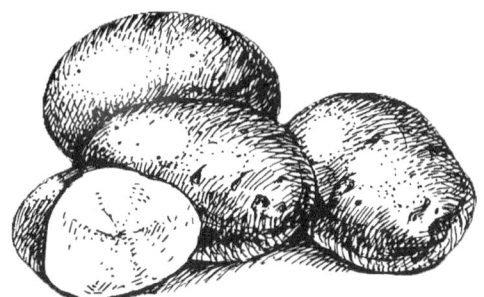

Manhattan Clam Chowder

The origins of Manhattan Clam Chowder are shrouded in lore. Some say this tomato-based chowder evolved from traditional New England milk-based chowders when Portuguese immigrants in Rhode Island added tomatoes. Others credit brothers William and James Winters whose Fulton Fish Market in Manhattan began selling tomato-based chowders after the brothers deemed milk to be too expensive. Either way this chowder is a light, refreshing alternative to its cream-laden New England cousin.

Ingredients

4 strips bacon, cut into 1/2" pieces
3/4 cup onion, finely diced
2 carrots, trimmed and halved lengthwise, halves sliced into 3/8" thick slices
3 ribs celery, sliced thinly into 3/8" thick slices
1 lb potatoes, cut into 1/2" cubes
1 tsp salt
1/4 tsp black pepper
1/2 tsp thyme, dried
1 tsp oregano, dried
1 tsp granulated garlic *
1/2 tsp hot red pepper flakes
2 tsp dried parsley flakes
1 8-oz bottle clam juice *
1/2 cup white wine (substitute water)
1 28-oz can tomatoes, diced or crushed (do not drain)
1 bay leaf
1 10-oz can baby clams, drained (reserve 1/2 cup liquid) and rinsed

* See *Tips* section

Cookware and Utensils

6-quart stockpot with lid
Vegetable peeler or paring knife (optional)
Small bowl
Mesh sieve
Liquid measuring cup (1-cup size or larger)

Instructions

1. Cut the bacon into 1/2-inch pieces. Add the bacon to the stockpot. Crisp the bacon on medium heat, stirring frequently.

2. Finely dice the onion. When the bacon is crisp add the onion to the stockpot. Stir to combine.

3. Scrub the carrots under running water and trim their ends. Halve each carrot lengthwise. Slice the halves into 3/8-inch thick slices. Add the carrots to the stockpot. Stir to combine.

4. Wash and trim the ends from the celery. Slice the celery into 3/8-inch thick slices. Add the celery to the stockpot. Stir to combine.

5. Scrub the potatoes under running water and peel them if desired. Cut the potatoes into 1/2-inch cubes. Add the potatoes to the stockpot. Stir to combine.

6. Add the salt, pepper, thyme, oregano, garlic, red pepper flakes, and the parsley to the small bowl. Stir to combine. Add the seasonings to the stockpot. Stir to coat the vegetables with the seasonings.

7. Add the clam juice, white wine (substitute water), tomatoes (do not drain), and the bay leaf to the stockpot. Stir to combine. Increase the heat to medium high until the mixture boils then reduce the heat to a gentle simmer.

8. Place a mesh sieve over the liquid measuring cup. Drain the clams through the mesh sieve reserving 1/2 cup of clam juice. Add the 1/2 cup of reserved clam juice to the stockpot. Stir to combine.

9. Rinse the clams with cold water and allow them to drain. Examine the clams for shell fragments. Remove foreign matter if necessary and discard.

10. Add the drained clams to the stockpot. Stir to combine. Cover the stockpot with the lid. Simmer the chowder until the potatoes and carrots pierce easily with the tines of a fork.

11. When the potatoes and carrots are tender remove the bay leaf. Serve the chowder hot.

Chipotle Shrimp and Avocado Soup

This recipe has its origins in the shrimp soups served on Fridays during the Lenten season when Mexican Catholics had to abstain from eating meat. Traditional Caldo de Camaron (Mexican Shrimp Soup) contains potatoes and carrots cooked in a tomato-based shrimp-infused broth. We've replaced the potatoes with convenient canned hominy and amped up the flavor with ground chipotle chili pepper, lime, and cilantro. Top the soup with some diced avocado which complements the smoky chipotle chili.

Ingredients

2 TBSP olive oil or vegetable oil
1/2 cup onion, finely diced
2 ribs celery, halved lengthwise,
  halves sliced into 3/8" thick slices
2 carrots, halved lengthwise,
  halves sliced into 3/8" thick slices
1/2 tsp salt
3/4 tsp granulated garlic *
1 tsp oregano, dried
  (use Mexican oregano if available)
1 tsp ground cumin
1 tsp ground chipotle chili
1 quart gluten-free chicken broth *
1 cup cilantro leaves
  (about 1 medium bunch)
2 TBSP lime juice (about 2 limes)
1 15-oz can tomatoes, diced or crushed
  (do not drain)
1 25-oz or 30-oz can hominy,
  rinsed and drained
12 oz frozen cooked shrimp,
  peeled, tails removed
1 avocado, peeled, pitted,
  and diced into 1/2" cubes

* See *Tips* section

Cookware and Utensils

6-quart stockpot with lid
Colander
Citrus juicer
Small serving bowl

Instructions

1. Add the oil to the stockpot. Finely dice the onion and add it to the stockpot. Stir to combine. Cook on medium low heat, stirring occasionally, until the onion is soft.

2. Trim the ends from the celery and halve each rib lengthwise. Slice each half into 3/8-inch thick slices. Add the celery to the stockpot. Stir to combine.

3. Scrub the carrots and trim their ends. Slice each carrot lengthwise. Slice each half into 3/8-inch thick slices. Add the carrots to the stockpot. Stir to combine.

4. Add the salt, garlic, oregano, cumin, and chipotle chili to the stockpot. Stir to coat the vegetables with the seasonings.

5. Add the chicken broth to the stockpot. Stir to combine. Cover the stockpot with the lid. Increase the heat to medium high until the broth boils then reduce the heat to a gentle simmer. Simmer, stirring occasionally, until the carrots pierce easily with the tines of a fork.

6. While the vegetables are simmering rinse and drain the cilantro in the colander. Remove the stems from the cilantro, reserving enough cilantro leaves to yield 1 cup. Juice the limes.

7. When the carrots pierce easily with the tines of a fork add the tomatoes (do not drain), cilantro, and 2 tablespoons of lime juice to the stockpot. Stir to combine.

8. Rinse and drain the hominy in the colander. Add the hominy to the stockpot. Stir to combine. Increase the heat to medium high until the soup boils then reduce the heat to a gentle simmer.

9. Rinse the shrimp with cold water in the colander and allow them to drain thoroughly. Remove any inedible tail material and discard. Add the shrimp to the stockpot. Simmer gently for 5 minutes to heat the shrimp. Do not overcook or the shrimp will become tough.

10. While the shrimp is heating peel and pit the avocado. Dice the avocado into 1/2-inch cubes and transfer it to the small serving bowl. Serve the soup hot with a spoonful of diced avocado on top.

Easy Cioppino

Cioppino (cho-PEE-no) is a stew of fish and shellfish in a chunky tomato broth that originated in San Francisco's Italian immigrant community. This mixed seafood stew was created when fishermen whose catch had not been successful wandered the port with a pot asking for contributions from fishermen who had been luckier that day.

Ingredients

2 TBSP olive oil or vegetable oil
1 cup onion, chopped
  (about 1/2 of a large onion)
3 cloves garlic, chopped
1 green bell pepper,
  seeded and diced into 1/2" pieces
1 tsp salt
1/4 tsp black pepper
1/2 tsp hot red pepper flakes
1/2 tsp thyme, dried
1 tsp oregano, dried
1/2 tsp basil, dried
2 tsp dried parsley flakes
1 8-oz bottle clam juice *
1/2 cup white wine (substitute water)
1 8-oz can tomato sauce
1 28-oz can tomatoes, diced or crushed
  (do not drain)
1 bay leaf
12 to 16 oz frozen shelled mixed
  seafood blend (shrimp, calamari,
  scallops, or other shellfish)
8 to 12 oz frozen firm white fish
  (cod, halibut, red snapper, haddock,
  pollock, or striped bass),
  skinned and deboned,
  cut into 1" pieces
1 lemon, juiced (about 2 TBSP juice)

* See *Tips* section

Instructions

1. If you will be making the (optional) garlic toast then preheat the oven to 300 degrees F.

2. Add the oil to the stockpot.

3. Chop the onion and the garlic. Add the onion and the garlic to the stockpot. Stir to coat the vegetables with the oil. Cook on medium heat, stirring frequently, until the onion is soft.

4. While the onion and garlic are cooking wash and seed the bell pepper. Dice the bell pepper into 1/2-inch pieces. Add the bell pepper to the stockpot. Stir to combine.

5. Add the salt, pepper, red pepper flakes, thyme, oregano, basil, and the parsley flakes to the small bowl. Stir to combine.

6. When the onions and the bell pepper are soft add the mixed seasonings to the stockpot. Stir to coat the vegetables with the seasonings.

7. Add the clam juice, white wine (substitute water), tomato sauce, canned tomatoes (do not drain), and the bay leaf to the stockpot. Stir to combine. Cover the stockpot with the lid. Increase the heat to medium high until the stew boils then reduce the heat to a gentle simmer.

8. Thaw the frozen shellfish by rinsing it in the colander with cold water. Remove and discard any shell fragments or inedible tail material. Allow the shellfish to drain thoroughly.

9. If making the (optional) garlic toast line a baking sheet with aluminum foil or parchment paper. Arrange the gluten-free bread in a single layer on the lined baking sheet.

10. Transfer the baking sheet to the oven. Toast the first side of the bread until slightly crunchy (about 10 minutes).

Continued

Easy Cioppino
- Continued -

Our simple version of this classic stew uses frozen seafood for those who are landlocked but feel free to substitute fresh seafood if you live near the ocean.

Optional Garlic Toast

8 slices gluten-free bread
2 TBSP olive oil
2 tsp granulated garlic *

* See *Tips* section

Cookware and Utensils

6-quart stockpot with lid
Small bowl
Colander
Metal baking sheet (optional)
Aluminum foil or parchment paper (optional)
Basting brush (optional)
Citrus juicer

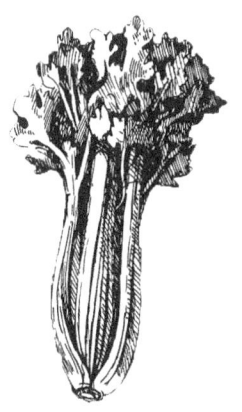

Instructions - continued

11. Remove the baking sheet from the oven. Flip each slice of bread. Baste the top sides of the bread slices with 2 tablespoons of olive oil. Sprinkle the bread slices lightly with 2 teaspoons of granulated garlic. Return the baking sheet to the oven. Toast the bread until the top side of the bread is light golden brown (about 10 minutes). Turn off the oven and keep the toast warm in the oven until serving time.

12. While the garlic toast is browning remove any skin or bones from the frozen fish and discard. Cut the fish into 1-inch pieces. Add the fish to the stockpot. Stir gently to combine. Cover the stockpot with the lid and simmer gently until the fish is opaque all the way through when cut with a knife. Stir minimally and do not overcook.

13. When the (optional) garlic toast is done add the drained shellfish to the stockpot. Stir gently to combine. Cover the stockpot with the lid. Increase the heat if necessary until the soup gently simmers. Adjust the heat to maintain a gentle simmer until the shellfish is completely cooked (opaque all the way through when cut with a knife). Simmer gently so that the shellfish does not become tough from overcooking.

14. While the shellfish is cooking juice the lemon. Add the lemon juice to the stockpot. Stir gently to combine.

15. When the fish and the shellfish are cooked all the way through remove the bay leaf. Serve the stew immediately with (optional) warm garlic toast.

Thai Shrimp and Noodle Soup

This quick and simple coconut milk-based shrimp soup gets a flavor kick from Thai chilis (also known as 'Bird's Eye' chilis). You can also substitute readily-available Serrano chili peppers. Be sure to select coconut milk processed without gluten-containing thickeners. Guar gum is commonly used as a thickener for coconut milk. Guar gum does not intentionally contain gluten.

Ingredients

1 quart gluten-free chicken broth *
1 cup water
1/2 tsp granulated garlic *
1/2 tsp ground ginger
1 tsp ground coriander
1 stalk lemongrass, trimmed and peeled, tender inner white bulb finely chopped (substitute 1/2 tsp dried lemongrass or omit this ingredient)
8 oz white button mushrooms, washed and sliced
7 to 8 oz Pad Thai-style rice noodles
2 green or red Thai chilis ('Bird's Eye' chilis) or 3 Serrano chili peppers, seeded and sliced into thin rounds
12 to 16 oz frozen cooked shrimp, peeled, tails removed
2 TBSP lime juice (about 2 limes)
1 TBSP brown sugar, firmly packed
2 TBSP Asian fish sauce
1 13.5-oz can coconut milk (without gluten-containing additives)

* See **Tips** section

Instructions

1. Add the chicken broth, water, garlic, ginger, and coriander to the stockpot. Stir to combine. Cover the stockpot with the lid. Heat on medium high heat until the broth begins to boil then reduce the heat to a gentle simmer.

2. While the broth is heating prepare the lemongrass (substitute 1/2 teaspoon of dried lemongrass or omit this ingredient). Trim the green top and the base of the lemongrass stalk, peel the tough dry outer layer of the bulb, and finely chop the tender inner white bulbous end of the stalk. Add the chopped lemongrass to the stockpot. Stir to combine.

3. Rinse the mushrooms in the colander and allow them to drain thoroughly. Slice the mushrooms. Add the mushrooms to the stockpot. Stir to combine. Cover the stockpot with the lid and continue simmering the broth while you prepare the rest of the ingredients.

4. Break the Pad Thai noodles in half and set them aside.

5. Prepare the (optional) condiments. Wash the basil leaves and slice them into thin ribbons. Transfer the basil to a small serving bowl. Wash and trim the ends of the green onions. Slice the green onions thinly into 1/4-inch thick slices. Transfer the sliced green onions to a small serving bowl. Rinse and drain the cilantro in the colander. Remove the cilantro leaves from the stems. Transfer the cilantro leaves to a small serving bowl. Refrigerate the condiments until serving time.

6. Prepare the chili peppers. You may want to wear disposable rubber gloves for this step to protect your hands, especially if you are a contact lens wearer as the chili oil can remain on your hands even after washing with soap. Rinse the Thai chili peppers (substitute Serrano peppers). Trim the stem end from the chilis and slit the chilis open lengthwise. Do not slice all the way through the chilis. Scoop out the seeds and discard. Slice the seeded chilis into thin rings. Add the sliced chilis to the stockpot. Stir to combine.

Continued

Thai Shrimp and Noodle Soup
- Continued -

Optional Condiments

1/4 cup fresh basil leaves,
  sliced into thin ribbons
1 bunch green onions,
  trimmed and sliced thinly
  into 1/4" thick slices
1 bunch cilantro, rinsed and destemmed

Cookware and Utensils

6-quart stockpot with lid
Colander
Citrus juicer
Small serving bowls
  for condiments (optional)

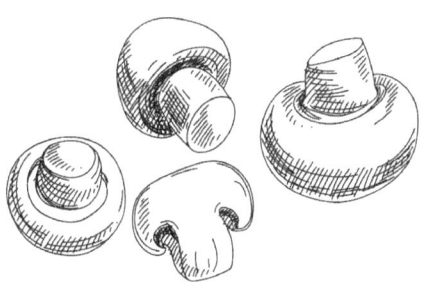

Instructions - continued

7. Rinse the frozen shrimp with cold water in the colander. Allow the shrimp to drain thoroughly. Remove and discard any inedible tail material.

8. Juice the limes. Reserve 2 tablespoons of lime juice.

9. When the mushrooms are soft add the broken Pad Thai noodles to the stockpot. Use a fork to gently separate the noodles until they are evenly distributed in the broth. Put the lid on the stockpot and cook the noodles on medium low heat until they are soft.

10. While the noodles are cooking measure 1 tablespoon of brown sugar by firmly packing the brown sugar into the measuring spoon and leveling the top. Set aside the brown sugar.

11. When the noodles are soft add the brown sugar, fish sauce, and 2 tablespoons of lime juice to the stockpot.

12. Shake the unopened can of coconut milk vigorously to disperse solids. Open the can of coconut milk and add it to the stockpot. Stir to combine.

13. Add the drained shrimp to the stockpot. Stir to combine. Adjust the heat to low and bring the soup to a gentle simmer. Allow the soup to simmer for a few minutes to heat the shrimp to serving temperature. Do not overcook or the shrimp will become tough.

14. Serve the soup immediately with (optional) condiments on the side.

Shrimp and Rice Gumbo

When Thomas Jefferson bought vast swaths of the United States from France's cash-strapped Napoleon Bonaparte via the Louisiana Purchase in 1803 he got the best deal since Dutch-American settlers bought the island of Manhattan for trinkets and beads. Not only did Jefferson get hundreds of thousands of miles of pristine land for 3 cents an acre, he got the culinary culture of the French, Spanish, and African settlers who gave us Louisiana's official state dish: gumbo.

Ingredients

1/4 cup olive oil or vegetable oil
12 oz frozen cut okra
1 cup onion, chopped
  (about 1/2 of a large onion)
1 green bell pepper,
  seeded and diced into 1/2" pieces
3 ribs celery, sliced into 3/8" thick slices
3/4 tsp salt
1/2 tsp black pepper
1/2 tsp thyme, dried
1 1/2 tsp oregano, dried
1/4 tsp hot red pepper flakes
1 1/2 tsp granulated garlic *
1/2 tsp cayenne pepper
1 15-oz can tomatoes, diced or crushed
  (do not drain)
1 8-oz can tomato sauce
1 quart gluten-free chicken broth *
2 bay leaves
1 cup converted (parboiled) rice **
12 to 16 oz frozen cooked shrimp,
  peeled, tails removed
  (substitute bay (salad) shrimp)

* See **Tips** section
** See **Converted Rice** section

Instructions

1. If you will be making the (optional) garlic toast then preheat the oven to 300 degrees F.

2. Add the oil and the okra to the stockpot. Stir to combine. Put the lid on the stockpot. Cook on medium heat, stirring occasionally, until the okra begins to soften.

3. While the okra is cooking chop the onion. Add the onion to the stockpot. Stir to combine.

4. Wash, seed, and dice the bell pepper into 1/2-inch pieces. Add the bell pepper to the stockpot. Stir to combine.

5. Wash and trim the ends from the celery. Slice the celery into 3/8-inch thick slices. Add the celery to the stockpot. Stir to combine. Put the lid on the stockpot and continue to cook, stirring occasionally, until the onion and bell pepper are soft.

6. Add the salt, pepper, thyme, oregano, red pepper flakes, garlic, and cayenne pepper to the small bowl. Stir to combine.

7. When the onion and bell pepper are soft add the seasonings to the stockpot. Stir to coat the vegetables with the seasonings.

8. Add the tomatoes (do not drain) and the tomato sauce to the stockpot. Stir to combine.

9. Add the chicken broth and the bay leaves to the stockpot. Stir to combine.

10. Add the converted (parboiled) rice to the stockpot. Stir to combine. Cover the stockpot with the lid. Increase the heat to medium high until the mixture boils then reduce the heat to a gentle simmer. Simmer gently, stirring occasionally, until the rice is fully cooked (about 25 minutes).

11. While the gumbo is simmering rinse the shrimp with cold water in the colander. Drain the shrimp thoroughly. Remove any inedible tail material and discard.

Continued

Shrimp and Rice Gumbo
- Continued -

Add extra cayenne if you like your gumbo spicy. To make this dish more economical use inexpensive bay shrimp (salad shrimp).

Optional Garlic Toast

8 slices gluten-free bread
2 TBSP olive oil
2 tsp granulated garlic *

* See *Tips* section

Cookware and Utensils

6-quart stockpot with lid
Small bowl
Colander
Metal baking sheet (optional)
Aluminum foil or parchment paper (optional)
Small bowl for olive oil (optional)
Basting brush (optional)

Instructions - continued

12. If making the optional garlic toast line a baking sheet with aluminum foil or parchment paper. Arrange the gluten-free bread in a single layer on the lined baking sheet.

13. Transfer the baking sheet to the oven. Toast the first side of the bread until slightly crunchy (about 10 minutes).

14. Remove the baking sheet from the oven. Flip each slice of bread. Baste the top sides of the bread slices with 2 tablespoons of olive oil. Sprinkle the bread slices lightly with 2 teaspoons of granulated garlic. Return the baking sheet to the oven. Toast the bread until the top side of the bread is light golden brown (about 10 minutes). Turn off the oven and keep the toast warm in the oven until serving time.

15. When the rice is fully cooked add the shrimp to the stockpot. Cover the stockpot with the lid. Simmer, covered, for 5 minutes to combine flavors and gently heat the shrimp to serving temperature (do not overcook or the shrimp will become tough).

16. After 5 minutes of simmering remove the bay leaves. Serve the gumbo hot with (optional) warm garlic bread.

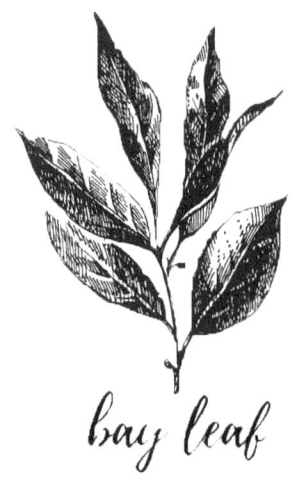
bay leaf

Seafood 167

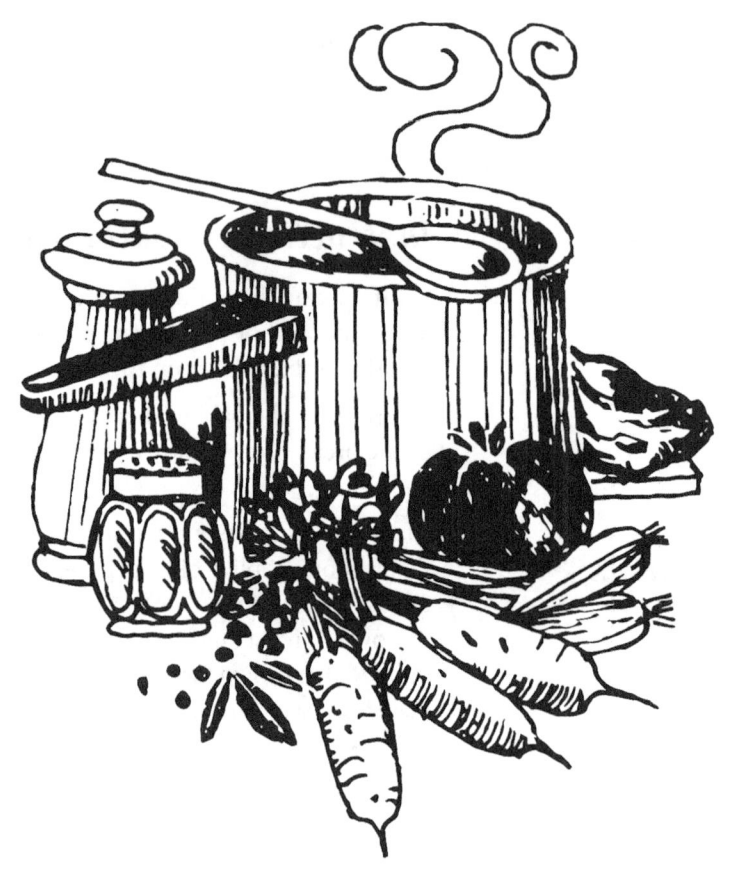

Vegetarian

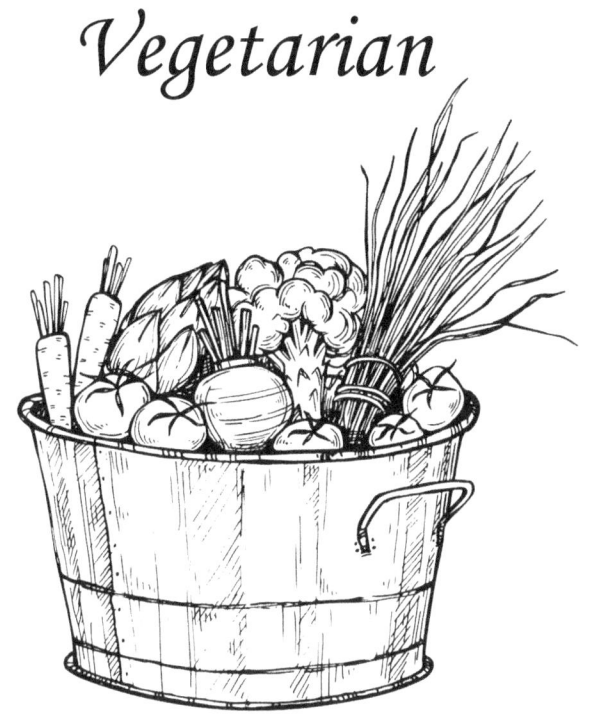

Meals in a Skillet

- 170 Pasta Primavera Skillet
- 171 Butternut Squash and Parmesan Skillet
- 172 Lentils with Kale and Sweet Potatoes

Soups and Stews

- 173 Provencal White Bean and Tomato Stew
- 174 Summertime Gazpacho
- 176 Sweet Potato and Black Bean Chili
- 177 Herbed Tomato Soup
- 178 Easy Ratatouille
- 180 Turkish Spinach and Lentil Stew
- 181 Savory Mushroom and Lentil Stew
- 182 Sweet Apple and Cabbage Stew
- 183 Winter Squash and Apple Soup
- 184 Italian Vegetable Stew
- 186 Curry Spiced Lentils

Pasta Primavera Skillet

Primavera means Spring in Italian, the time when the garden is abundant with slender shoots of asparagus, tender green peas, and the first sprigs of basil. This skillet can be enjoyed year round as it makes use of frozen vegetables but feel free to substitute fresh vegetables if available. Just add them a little sooner so that they are cooked tender crisp by the time the pasta is done.

Ingredients

8 to 10 oz frozen asparagus spears, thawed and cut into 2" lengths
3/4 cup frozen peas
1/2 cup onion, finely diced
3 TBSP butter
1 tsp salt
1/4 tsp black pepper
1/2 tsp thyme, dried
1/4 tsp tarragon, dried
1 tsp basil, dried
  (substitute 2 tablespoons fresh basil sliced into thin ribbons)
1 tsp granulated garlic *
1 cup water, heated
2 cups milk *
8 oz gluten-free pasta **
3/4 cup grated Parmesan cheese *
1 pint cherry tomatoes, rinsed and cut in half

* See *Tips* section
** See *Measuring Pasta* section

Cookware and Utensils

12-inch skillet with lid
Microwave-safe liquid measuring cup
  (1-cup size or larger)
Shredder/grater
  (if not using pre-grated cheese)
Colander

Instructions

1. Remove the frozen asparagus from the freezer. Measure 3/4 cup of frozen peas. Thaw the asparagus and the peas on the countertop while preparing the pasta.

2. Finely dice the onion.

3. Add the butter and the onion to the skillet. Heat on low heat until the onion is soft. Stir occasionally.

4. Add the salt, pepper, thyme, tarragon, basil, and garlic to the onion. Stir to combine.

5. Microwave 1 cup of water on high power for 1 minute.

6. Add the hot water and the milk to the skillet. Stir to combine.

7. Add the gluten-free pasta to the skillet. Stir to combine. Cover the skillet with the lid. Increase the heat to medium high until the mixture boils then reduce the heat to a gentle simmer.

8. Most gluten-free pastas cook in 7 to 12 minutes. Stir the mixture frequently, checking every 3 to 4 minutes until the water is almost all absorbed and the pasta is nearly done.

9. While the pasta is cooking grate the Parmesan cheese (if not using pre-grated cheese).

10. Rinse the cherry tomatoes in the colander and allow them to drain. Cut each cherry tomato in half.

11. If necessary cut the asparagus spears into 2-inch lengths.

12. When the pasta is nearly cooked to the desired doneness (not all the water will be absorbed) stir in the peas and asparagus. Cover the skillet with the lid and heat for a few minutes until the pasta is fully cooked and the vegetables are tender crisp.

13. Stir in the grated Parmesan cheese. Cover the skillet with the lid. Turn off the heat and allow the cheese to melt. Stir again to combine.

14. Add the cherry tomatoes to the skillet. Stir gently to combine. Serve immediately.

Butternut Squash and Parmesan Skillet

This skillet is a healthier alternative to standard 'macaroni and cheese' dishes. Use water or vegetable broth for a vegetarian option. Those who eat meat in their diet can substitute chicken broth for a savory flavor.

Ingredients

10 to 12 oz frozen puréed butternut squash or other winter squash
1 1/2 cups onion, chopped
3 TBSP butter
1 TBSP brown sugar, firmly packed
1 tsp salt
1/4 tsp black pepper
1/2 tsp rosemary, dried
1/4 tsp thyme, dried
1/4 tsp ground nutmeg
1/4 tsp ground sage
1 1/4 cups water, heated
  (substitute gluten-free vegetable broth or gluten-free chicken broth *)
2 cups milk *
8 oz gluten-free pasta **
1 cup grated Parmesan cheese *

* See *Tips* section
** See *Measuring Pasta* section

Cookware and Utensils

Microwave-safe dish to defrost frozen squash
12-inch skillet with lid
Microwave-safe liquid measuring cup (2-cup size or larger)
Shredder/grater (if not using pre-grated cheese)

Instructions

1. Transfer the puréed frozen squash to a microwave-safe dish and cover with a clean paper towel to reduce splatter inside the microwave. Defrost on low power for 3 minutes or until the squash is nearly thawed. Remove the squash from the microwave and continue thawing on the countertop until you are ready to add it to the skillet.

2. Chop the onion.

3. Add the butter and the onion to the skillet. Cook on low heat until the onion is soft, stirring frequently.

4. Add the thawed squash to the skillet. Stir to combine.

5. Measure the brown sugar by firmly packing it into the measuring spoon and leveling the top of the spoon. Add the salt, pepper, rosemary, thyme, nutmeg, sage, and the brown sugar to the squash and onion mixture. Stir to combine.

6. Microwave 1 1/4 cups of water on high power for 1 minute and 30 seconds. Gluten-free vegetable broth or gluten-free chicken broth may be substituted for added flavor.

7. Add the hot water (or broth) and the milk to the squash and onion mixture. Stir to combine.

8. Add the gluten free pasta to the skillet. Stir to combine. Cover the skillet with the lid. Increase the heat to medium high until the mixture boils then reduce the heat to a gentle simmer. It will take longer for the pasta to cook in this recipe because of the puréed squash in the cooking liquid. Stir the mixture frequently, checking every 3 to 4 minutes until the pasta is cooked to your taste.

9. While the pasta is cooking grate the Parmesan cheese (if not using pre-grated cheese).

10. When the pasta is cooked to the desired doneness stir in the grated Parmesan cheese. Cover the skillet with the lid. Reduce the heat to low and heat for a few minutes to melt the cheese. Stir to combine. Serve immediately.

Lentils with Kale and Sweet Potatoes

Lentils are a staple of Middle Eastern, Indian, and North African cuisine because they cook quickly and provide a much-needed source of protein. This vegan recipe pairs lentils with crunchy kale (high in calcium) and tender sweet potatoes (a good source of Vitamin A). If you like your food spicy then add more hot red pepper flakes.

Ingredients

1 cup onion, chopped
  (about 1/2 of a large onion)
2 TBSP olive oil or vegetable oil
1 lb sweet potatoes or yams,
  peeled and cut into 1/2" cubes
3/4 tsp salt
1/4 tsp black pepper
1/4 tsp hot red pepper flakes
1 tsp ground cumin
1 tsp ground coriander
1 tsp granulated garlic *
2 cups gluten-free vegetable broth *
  (substitute water)
2 tsp red wine vinegar
1 bay leaf
1 cup lentils, dried
10 to 12 oz kale, washed, ribs and stems
  removed, torn in large pieces
  (substitute pre-washed and cut kale)

* See *Tips* section

Cookware and Utensils

12-inch skillet with lid
Vegetable peeler or paring knife
Small bowl
Colander

Instructions

1. Chop the onion.

2. Add the onion and the oil to the skillet. Stir to combine. Heat on low heat, stirring occasionally, until the onion is soft.

3. While the onion is cooking peel and dice the sweet potatoes or yams into 1/2-inch cubes. Add the sweet potatoes or yams to the onion. Stir to combine.

4. Measure the salt, black pepper, red pepper flakes, cumin, coriander, and garlic into a small bowl. Stir to combine.

5. When the onion is soft sprinkle the seasonings over the onion and sweet potato mixture. Stir to coat the vegetables with the seasonings.

6. Add the vegetable broth (substitute water), red wine vinegar, and the bay leaf to the skillet. Stir to combine.

7. Rinse the lentils in the colander and allow them to drain completely. Inspect the lentils carefully for rocks or other foreign matter that could chip a tooth. Discard foreign matter if necessary. Add the rinsed lentils to the skillet. Stir to combine.

8. Cover the skillet with the lid. Increase the heat to medium high until the liquid boils then reduce the heat to a gentle simmer.

9. Wash, de-stem, and tear the kale into large pieces (if not using pre-washed and cut kale).

10. When the lentils begin to soften layer the kale in an even layer over the lentil and vegetable mixture. Cover the skillet with the lid.

11. Simmer, covered, on low heat until the lentils are tender but still firm and the sweet potatoes pierce easily with the tines of a fork. Stir to combine the kale into the lentils and sweet potatoes. Remove the bay leaf. Serve immediately.

Provencal White Bean and Tomato Stew

This vegetarian stew is based on traditional French Provencal stews that feature tender white beans, tomatoes, savory herbs, and olive oil - all staples of Provencal cooking. Frozen spinach has been added for extra nutrition but feel free to substitute fresh spinach if it's in season. Rinse and drain the spinach well then add it after the onion is soft.

Ingredients

10 to 12 oz frozen chopped spinach
1 cup onion, chopped
  (about 1/2 of a large onion)
3 TBSP olive oil or vegetable oil
1/2 cup water
1 tsp salt
1/4 tsp black pepper
1/2 tsp rosemary, dried
1/2 tsp thyme, dried
1/2 tsp sage, dried
1 tsp granulated garlic *
1 15-oz can diced tomatoes
  (do not drain) or 2 large tomatoes,
  cut into 1/2" cubes
3 15-oz cans white beans
  (Cannellini, Great Northern, Navy, or
  other white beans), rinsed and drained

* See *Tips* section

Cookware and Utensils

6-quart stockpot with lid
Colander

Instructions

1. Remove the frozen chopped spinach from the freezer and transfer it to the countertop to thaw.

2. Chop the onion.

3. Add the onion and the oil to the stockpot. Stir to combine. Heat on medium heat, stirring occasionally, until the onion is soft.

4. When the onion is soft add the water and the frozen chopped spinach to the stockpot. Stir to combine. Cover the stockpot with the lid and continue cooking on medium heat until the spinach has thawed. Stir occasionally.

5. Add the salt, pepper, rosemary, thyme, sage, and garlic to the onion and spinach mixture. Stir to combine.

6. If using canned tomatoes add them to the stockpot (do not drain the tomatoes). If using fresh tomatoes cut them into 1/2-inch cubes and add them to the stockpot. Stir to combine. Heat on medium heat until the stew begins to boil then reduce the heat to a gentle simmer.

7. While the stew is simmering rinse the beans in the colander and allow them to drain thoroughly.

8. Add the drained beans to the stockpot. Stir gently to combine. Cover the stockpot with the lid. Simmer the stew on low heat for 10 minutes to combine flavors. Serve hot.

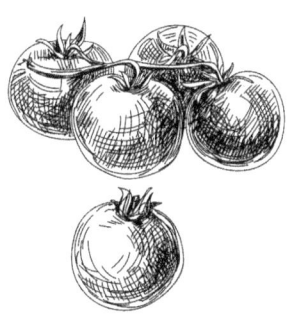

Summertime Gazpacho

Summer is a glorious time of year when the garden and markets are abundant with fresh tomatoes, cucumbers, and bell peppers. Originally from Spain and Portugal, Gazpacho is a chilled soup that makes good use of these abundant summertime ingredients and is perfect for a light dinner on a hot summer evening.

Ingredients

3 cups unflavored tomato juice
3/4 tsp salt
1/4 tsp black pepper
1/2 tsp hot red pepper flakes
1 TBSP olive oil or vegetable oil
1 lemon, juiced (about 2 TBSP juice)
2 garlic cloves, finely chopped
1 cup onion, finely diced
 (substitute red onion for more flavor)
1 green bell pepper,
 seeded and diced into 1/2" pieces
3 ribs celery, halved lengthwise,
 halves sliced thinly into 3/8" thick slices
1 cucumber, peeled, seeds scooped,
 cut into 3/8" cubes
1 1/2 lbs very ripe tomatoes,
 cut into 3/8" cubes
3 TBSP fresh basil, coarsely chopped
 (substitute 3/4 tsp dried basil)

Instructions

1. Add the tomato juice, salt, pepper, red pepper flakes, and the oil to a non-metallic bowl. Stir to combine.

2. Juice the lemon. Add the lemon juice to the bowl. Stir to combine.

3. Finely chop the garlic. Add the garlic to the bowl. Stir to combine.

4. Finely dice the onion. Add the onion to the bowl. Stir to combine.

5. Seed and dice the bell pepper into 1/2-inch pieces. Add the bell pepper to the bowl. Stir to combine.

6. Trim the ends of the celery and slice each rib in half lengthwise. Slice the celery thinly into 3/8-inch thick slices. Add the celery to the bowl. Stir to combine.

7. Peel the cucumber. Scoop out any large seeds with a spoon. Cut the seeded cucumber into 3/8-inch cubes. Add the cucumber to the bowl. Stir to combine.

8. Wash the tomatoes and cut off the blossom end. Cut the tomatoes into 3/8-inch cubes. Add the tomatoes to the bowl. Stir to combine.

9. Wash and coarsely chop enough basil leaves to yield 3 tablespoons (substitute 3/4 teaspoon dried basil). Add the basil to the bowl. Stir to combine.

10. Cover the bowl with plastic wrap and refrigerate until well chilled (3-4 hours). Served chilled.

Continued

Summertime Gazpacho
- Continued -

Make this chunky soup in the afternoon and refrigerate until well chilled. After the sun goes down light a few candles, open a bottle of red wine, and pair this chilled soup with (optional) gluten-free garlic toast for a simple al fresco meal.

Optional Garlic Toast

8 slices gluten-free bread
2 TBSP olive oil
2 tsp granulated garlic *

* See *Tips* section

Cookware and Utensils

Non-metallic bowl, 3-quart size
Citrus juicer
Vegetable peeler or paring knife
Metal baking sheet (optional)
Aluminum foil or parchment paper
 (optional)
Small bowl for olive oil (optional)
Basting brush (optional)

Instructions - Garlic Toast

1. Preheat the oven to 300 degrees F.

2. Line a baking sheet with aluminum foil or parchment paper. Arrange the gluten-free bread in a single layer on the lined baking sheet.

3. Transfer the baking sheet to the oven. Toast the first side of the bread until slightly crunchy (about 10 minutes).

4. Remove the baking sheet from the oven. Flip each slice of bread. Baste the top sides of the bread slices with 2 tablespoons of olive oil. Sprinkle the bread slices lightly with 2 teaspoons of granulated garlic.

5. Return the baking sheet to the oven. Toast the bread until the top side of the bread is light golden brown (about 10 minutes). Turn off the oven and keep the toast warm in the oven until serving time.

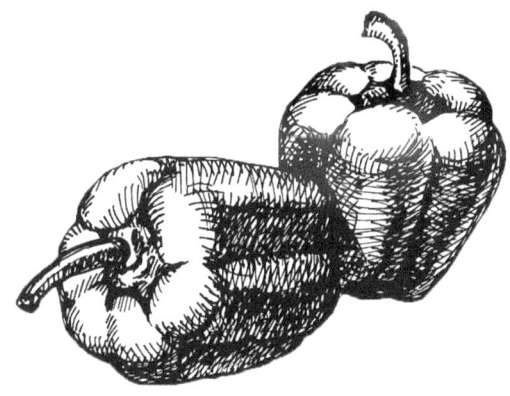

Sweet Potato and Black Bean Chili

This sweet and spicy vegetarian chili cooks up quick and is perfect for a light meal or as an accompaniment to grilled portobello mushrooms or grilled meats. It uses ground chipotle chili that has a smoky flavor that complements the black beans. Garnish this chili with diced avocado or corn tortilla chips if desired.

Ingredients

2 TBSP vegetable oil
1 cup onion, chopped
  (about 1/2 of large onion)
1 red bell pepper, seeded and diced
  into 1/2" pieces
1 large sweet potato or yam,
  peeled and cut into 1/2" cubes
1/4 tsp salt
1 tsp sugar
1 tsp ground cumin
1 tsp granulated garlic *
1 tsp ground chipotle chili
1 TBSP chili powder *
1 cup water
1 15-oz can tomatoes, diced or crushed
  (do not drain)
2 15-oz cans black beans,
  rinsed and drained
1 cup cilantro leaves (optional
  – about 1 medium bunch)

* See **Tips** section

Optional Garnishes

1 avocado, peeled, pit removed,
  diced into 1/2" cubes
Corn chips or corn tortilla chips

Cookware and Utensils

6-quart stockpot with lid
Vegetable peeler or paring knife
Colander

Instructions

1. Add the oil to the stockpot.

2. Chop the onion and add it to the stockpot. Stir to combine. Cook on medium low heat, stirring occasionally, until the onion is soft.

3. Seed and dice the bell pepper into 1/2-inch pieces. When the onion is soft add the bell pepper to the stockpot. Stir to combine.

4. Peel the sweet potato (or yam) and cut it into 1/2-inch cubes. Add the sweet potato to the stockpot. Stir to combine.

5. Add the salt, sugar, cumin, garlic, chipotle chili, and chili powder to the stockpot. Stir to coat the vegetables with the seasonings.

6. Add 1 cup of water to the stockpot. Stir to combine. Cover the stockpot with the lid. Increase the heat to medium high until the mixture boils then reduce the heat to a gentle simmer. Simmer covered for 10 to 15 minutes until the sweet potatoes pierce easily with the tines of a fork. Stir occasionally.

7. When the sweet potatoes are tender add the tomatoes to the stockpot (do not drain). Stir to combine.

8. Rinse and drain the beans in the colander. Add the beans to the stockpot. Stir to combine. Cover the stockpot with the lid. Increase the heat to medium high until the chili boils then reduce the heat to a gentle simmer. Simmer covered for 15 minutes to combine flavors. Stir occasionally.

9. If adding the optional cilantro rinse and drain the cilantro in the colander. Remove the stems from enough cilantro leaves to yield 1 cup. Add the cilantro to the stockpot. Stir to combine. Cover the stockpot with the lid and continue simmering for the remainder of the 15 minute interval to combine flavors.

10. If serving the chili with the optional avocado garnish then peel and pit the avocado. Dice the avocado into 1/2-inch cubes.

11. Serve the chili hot with (optional) diced avocado, corn chips, or corn tortilla chips.

Herbed Tomato Soup

One of the great joys of life is a hot bowl of creamy tomato soup with a gluten-free grilled cheese sandwich. For those who must avoid gluten this can be a problem because so many of the cream-based tomato soups contain wheat flour as a thickener. This easy soup is quick and uses herbs, shallots, and red wine for a savory piquant flavor that pairs well with a sharp Cheddar or a nutty Gouda cheese. For a kid-friendly version substitute finely diced onion for the shallots and omit the red wine.

Ingredients

1 TBSP vegetable oil
2/3 cup shallots, finely diced
  (about 2 large shallots
   – substitute 1/2 cup
  finely diced onion)
1/2 tsp salt
1/4 tsp black pepper
1/2 tsp thyme, dried
1/4 tsp basil, dried
1 15-oz can tomato sauce
  (substitute two 8-oz cans
  tomato sauce)
1/2 cup red wine (optional)
1 1/3 cups half-and-half

Cookware and Utensils

2-quart saucepan with lid
  (or larger)

Instructions

1. Add the oil to the saucepan.

2. Finely dice the shallots (or onion) and add them to the saucepan. Stir to combine. Cook the shallots on medium low heat, stirring occasionally, until the shallots are soft.

3. When the shallots are soft add the salt, pepper, thyme, and basil to the saucepan. Stir to combine.

4. Add the tomato sauce to the saucepan. Stir to combine.

5. Add the (optional) red wine to the saucepan. Stir to combine. Heat the soup on medium low heat to a gentle simmer.

6. When the soup is gently simmering add the half-and-half to the saucepan. Stir to combine. Reduce the heat to low and cook, stirring occasionally, until the soup is at serving temperature. Do not boil the soup or the cream will separate. Serve immediately.

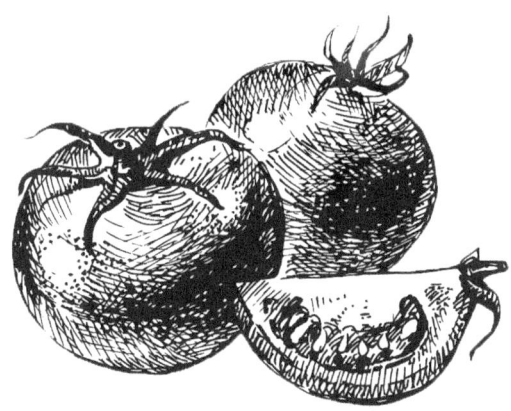

Easy Ratatouille

In the summer, gardens in the Provence region of southern France offer up a wealth of fresh vegetables that are made into a stew called Ratatouille ('rat-uh-TOO-ee'). This chunky stew of eggplant, zucchini, tomatoes, and bell peppers is equally delicious served warm as a main course or chilled as an appetizer.

Ingredients

3 TBSP olive oil or vegetable oil
1 1/2 cups onion, sliced into crescents (about 1/2 of a large onion)
3 cloves garlic, finely chopped
1 bell pepper (green, red, orange, or yellow), seeded and cut into strips, strips halved
1 zucchini or yellow summer squash, ends trimmed, halved lengthwise, halves sliced into 3/8" thick slices
1 large eggplant, peeled and cut into 1" cubes
1 1/2 lbs very ripe tomatoes, cut into 1" cubes
1 tsp salt
1/4 tsp black pepper
1 tsp thyme, dried
1/2 tsp oregano, dried
1/4 tsp hot red pepper flakes
1/2 cup red wine (substitute water)
1 bay leaf
1/4 cup fresh basil leaves, washed and sliced into ribbons (substitute 1 tsp dried basil)

Instructions

1. If you will be making the (optional) garlic toast then preheat the oven to 300 degrees F.

2. Add the oil to the stockpot.

3. Slice the onion into crescents. Add the onion to the stockpot.

4. Finely chop the garlic. Add the garlic to the stockpot. Stir to combine. Cook the onion and garlic on medium low heat, stirring occasionally.

5. Wash and seed the bell pepper. Cut the bell pepper into strips then halve each strip. Add the bell pepper to the stockpot. Stir to combine.

6. Wash and trim the ends of the zucchini or summer squash. Slice the zucchini or summer squash in half lengthwise then slice each half into 3/8-inch thick slices. Add the zucchini or summer squash to the stockpot. Stir to combine.

7. Wash and peel the eggplant. Cut the eggplant into 1-inch cubes. Add the eggplant to the stockpot. Stir to combine. Cover the stockpot with the lid to steam the vegetables as they cook.

8. Wash the tomatoes and cut off the blossom end. Cut the tomatoes into 1-inch cubes. Add the tomatoes to the stockpot. Stir to combine.

9. Add the salt, pepper, thyme, oregano, and red pepper flakes to the stockpot. Stir to combine.

10. Add the red wine (substitute water) and the bay leaf to the stockpot. Stir to combine.

11. Wash the basil and slice it into thin ribbons to yield 1/4 cup (substitute 1 tsp dried basil). Add the basil to the stockpot. Stir to combine. Cover the stockpot with the lid and adjust the heat until the stew simmers gently. Simmer for 30 minutes. Stir occasionally.

Continued

Easy Ratatouille
- Continued -

Pair this stew with the optional gluten-free garlic toast for a complete and satisfying meal.

Optional Garlic Toast

8 slices gluten-free bread
2 TBSP olive oil
2 tsp granulated garlic *

* See *Tips* section

Cookware and Utensils

6-quart stockpot with lid
Vegetable peeler or paring knife
Metal baking sheet (optional)
Aluminum foil or parchment paper (optional)
Small bowl for olive oil (optional)
Basting brush (optional)

Instructions - continued

12. If making the optional garlic toast line a baking sheet with aluminum foil or parchment paper. Arrange the gluten-free bread in a single layer on the lined baking sheet.

13. Transfer the baking sheet to the oven. Toast the first side of the bread until slightly crunchy (about 10 minutes).

14. Remove the baking sheet from the oven. Flip each slice of bread. Baste the top sides of the bread slices with 2 tablespoons of olive oil. Sprinkle the bread slices lightly with 2 teaspoons of granulated garlic. Return the baking sheet to the oven. Toast the bread until the top side of the bread is light golden brown (about 10 minutes). Turn off the oven and keep the toast warm in the oven until serving time.

15. After the stew has simmered for 30 minutes check the eggplant for doneness. If the eggplant is not soft continue simmering for an additional 10 minutes or until the eggplant is soft.

16. When the eggplant is soft remove the bay leaf. Serve the stew hot with (optional) warm garlic toast. This stew can also be refrigerated overnight and served as a chilled appetizer.

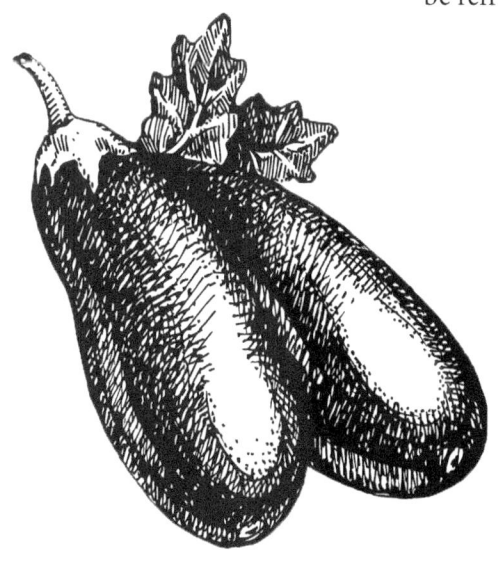

Turkish Spinach and Lentil Stew

This simple and surprisingly delicious stew is based on Turkish spinach and lentil soups and an Armenian soup, Shomini Aboor, that is served during the 40-day Lenten season when Armenian Christians must practice a vegan diet. Traditional Shomini Aboor contains bulgur wheat (cracked wheat) which contains gluten. This recipe substitutes buckwheat which, despite its name, is gluten-free. Those who eat meat can substitute chicken broth for the water to add a savory flavor.

Ingredients

8 cups water (substitute 1 quart gluten-free chicken broth * + 4 cups water)
1 cup lentils (about 8 oz), rinsed and drained
1 tsp basil, dried (substitute 2 TBSP fresh basil, coarsely chopped)
1 cup buckwheat (about 7 oz), rinsed and drained
2 tsp salt
1 1/2 tsp granulated garlic *
1 28-oz can tomatoes, crushed or diced (do not drain)
1 15-oz can tomato sauce (substitute two 8-oz cans tomato sauce)
10 oz frozen spinach (substitute 8 to 10 oz fresh spinach, washed and coarsely chopped)

* See *Tips* section

Cookware and Utensils

6-quart stockpot with lid
Mesh sieve

Instructions

1. Add 8 cups of water to the stockpot (you may substitute 1 quart of gluten-free chicken broth plus 4 cups of water). Cover the stockpot with the lid. Heat the water or broth on medium high heat until it boils then reduce the heat to a gentle simmer.

2. While the water or broth is heating rinse the lentils under running water in a mesh sieve. Inspect the lentils carefully for rocks or other foreign matter that could chip a tooth. Discard foreign matter if necessary. Drain the lentils thoroughly.

3. When the water or broth begins to boil add the lentils to the stockpot. Stir to combine. Cover the stockpot with the lid. Adjust the heat to maintain a gentle simmer. Simmer the lentils, covered, for 30 minutes. Stir occasionally.

4. If you will be using fresh basil wash and coarsely chop enough basil leaves to yield 2 tablespoons.

5. After the lentils have simmered for 30 minutes rinse the buckwheat under running water in a mesh sieve. Drain the buckwheat and add it to the stockpot. Stir to combine.

6. Add the salt, garlic, basil, tomatoes (do not drain), and the tomato sauce to the stockpot. Stir to combine.

7. Add the spinach to the stockpot. Stir to combine. If using fresh spinach which is bulky you may need to add the spinach leaves in portions, allowing the first portion to wilt before adding additional portions. This recipe will almost completely fill the 6-quart stockpot so do not overfill.

8. When all of the spinach has been added to the stockpot stir to combine. Cover the stockpot with the lid. Increase the heat to medium high until the stew boils then reduce the heat to a gentle simmer.

9. Simmer the stew for 20 to 25 minutes, stirring occasionally until the lentils are tender but still firm and not yet mushy. The buckwheat will be soft and slightly chewy.

10. Serve the stew hot. This recipe makes a big pot of stew so you will have leftovers. Refrigerate leftovers. To reheat leftovers, add a few tablespoons of water as the stew will thicken during refrigeration.

Savory Mushroom and Lentil Stew

Mushrooms, herbs, and lots of garlic give this vegetarian stew its savory flavor. Lentils, potatoes, and carrots make it a satisfying one-pot meal. For a more intense mushroom flavor use cremini mushrooms (baby portobello mushrooms) instead of white button mushrooms. This stew can be made vegan by substituting rice milk or soy milk for the half-and-half.

Ingredients

3 TBSP vegetable oil
1 1/2 cups onion, chopped
8 oz mushrooms, white button or
  cremini (baby portobello mushrooms),
  washed and sliced
1 1/2 tsp salt
1/4 tsp black pepper
1 tsp thyme, dried
1/2 tsp rosemary, dried
1/2 tsp marjoram, dried
1/4 tsp hot red pepper flakes
2 tsp granulated garlic *
3 cups water
1/2 cup white wine (substitute water)
3 TBSP wheat-free Tamari Sauce *
1 bay leaf
1 cup lentils (about 8 oz),
  rinsed and drained
3 carrots, trimmed and halved
  lengthwise, halves sliced
  into 3/8" thick slices
1 lb potatoes,
  scrubbed and cut into 1/2" cubes
1/2 cup half-and-half
  (substitute rice milk or soy milk)

* See *Tips* section

Cookware and Utensils

6-quart stockpot with lid
Colander
Mesh sieve

Instructions

1. Add the oil to the stockpot. Chop the onion and add it to the stockpot. Stir to combine. Cook on medium low heat until the onion is soft. Stir occasionally.

2. Rinse the mushrooms in the colander and allow them to drain thoroughly. Slice the mushrooms. When the onion is soft add the mushrooms to the stockpot. Stir to combine. Cover the stockpot with the lid. Continue cooking on medium low heat until the mushrooms are soft. Stir occasionally.

3. When the mushrooms are soft add the salt, pepper, thyme, rosemary, marjoram, red pepper flakes, and garlic to the stockpot. Stir to coat the mushroom and onion mixture with the seasonings.

4. Add 3 cups of water, the white wine (you may substitute water), the Tamari Sauce, and the bay leaf to the stockpot. Stir to combine.

5. Rinse the lentils in a mesh sieve. Inspect the lentils carefully for rocks or other foreign matter that could chip a tooth. Discard foreign matter if necessary. Drain the lentils and add them to the stockpot. Stir to combine. Cover the stockpot with the lid. Increase the heat to medium high until the stew boils then reduce the heat to a gentle simmer.

6. Scrub the carrots under running water, trim their ends, and halve them lengthwise. Slice each half into 3/8-inch thick slices. Add the carrots to the stockpot. Stir to combine.

7. Scrub the potatoes under running water. Cut the potatoes into 1/2-inch cubes. Add the potatoes to the stockpot. Stir to combine. Cover the stockpot with the lid and simmer the stew for 25 minutes. Stir occasionally.

8. After the stew has simmered for 25 minutes test the lentils for doneness. The lentils are fully cooked when they are tender but still firm and not yet mushy. If the lentils are not completely cooked simmer for an additional 10 minutes then test again.

9. When the lentils are tender remove the bay leaf. Add the half-and-half to the stockpot (substitute rice milk or soy milk). Stir to combine. Serve hot.

Sweet Apple and Cabbage Stew

Cabbage and apple cider vinegar are both well known for their ability to detoxify the body. This recipe pairs the beneficial properties of these foods with apples and sweet onions for a healthy, flavorful vegetarian meal. Try Walla Walla, Vidalia, or Maui onions which are sweet varieties that are easy to find at your grocer. Those who eat meat in their diet can add the optional diced ham if desired.

Ingredients

2 TBSP vegetable oil
1 1/2 cups sweet onion,
  sliced into crescents
  (about 1/2 of a large onion)
3 large apples, peeled, cored,
  and thinly sliced
12 oz ham, diced into 1/2" cubes *
  (optional)
1/2 tsp salt
1/4 tsp pepper
2 cups apple cider (substitute apple juice)
2 tsp apple cider vinegar
1 small head green cabbage
  (about 1 1/2 lbs), cored, quartered,
  and thinly sliced

* See *Tips* section

Cookware and Utensils

6-quart stockpot with lid
Paring knife

Instructions

1. Add the oil to the stockpot.

2. Slice the onion into crescents 1/2-inch thick. Add the onion to the stockpot. Cook the onion on medium heat until it is soft.

3. While the onion is cooking peel, core, and slice the apples into 3/8-inch thick slices. Add the apples to the stockpot. Stir to combine.

4. If you will be adding the optional ham then dice the ham into 1/2-inch cubes. Add the diced ham to the stockpot. Stir to combine.

5. Add the salt, pepper, apple cider (substitute apple juice), and the apple cider vinegar to the stockpot. Stir to combine.

6. Remove the tough outer leaves of the cabbage. Cut the hard center core from the cabbage. Slice the cabbage into quarters. Slice each quarter thinly into 3/8-inch thick strips.

7. Add the sliced cabbage to the stockpot. Stir to combine. Cover the stockpot with the lid. Increase the heat to medium high until the stew boils then reduce the heat to a gentle simmer.

8. Simmer for 15 to 20 minutes, stirring occasionally, until the cabbage and apples are tender. Serve the stew hot.

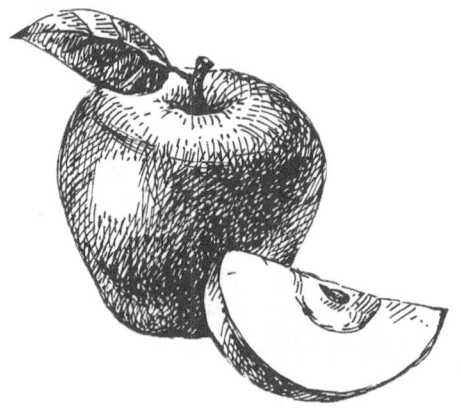

Winter Squash and Apple Soup

This savory Winter Squash and Apple Soup is made quick and easy through the use of frozen puréed butternut squash that requires no time-consuming peeling and seeding. If frozen puréed squash is not available you can substitute canned puréed pumpkin.

Ingredients

10 to 12 oz frozen puréed squash
  (substitute one 15-oz can
  puréed pumpkin)
1 TBSP vegetable oil
1 1/2 cups onion, chopped
2 apples, peeled, cored,
  and diced into 3/8" cubes
1 tsp salt
1/4 tsp black pepper
1/4 tsp ground nutmeg
1 1/4 tsp ground ginger
1/4 tsp ground sage
3/4 tsp granulated garlic *
2 TBSP brown sugar, packed
2 cups apple juice
1 1/2 cups half-and-half

* See *Tips* section

Optional Garnish

8 oz Gouda or sharp Cheddar cheese,
  cut into wedges or slices

Cookware and Utensils

6-quart stockpot with lid
Vegetable peeler or paring knife

Instructions

1. Transfer the frozen squash to the countertop to thaw while you are preparing the soup.

2. If you will be serving the (optional) Gouda or Cheddar cheese then for best flavor cut the cheese into wedges or slices, arrange on a serving tray, cover with plastic wrap, and let the cheese come to room temperature before serving.

3. Add the oil to the stockpot.

4. Chop the onion. Add the onion to the stockpot. Stir to coat the onion with the oil. Cook on medium low heat, stirring occasionally.

5. While the onion is cooking peel and core the apples. Dice the apples into small cubes 3/8-inch in size. Add the apples to the stockpot. Stir to combine. Cover the stockpot with the lid. Increase the heat to medium and cook, stirring occasionally, until the onion and apples are soft.

6. When the onion and the apples are soft add the salt, pepper, nutmeg, ginger, sage, and garlic to the stockpot. Stir to combine.

7. Measure 2 tablespoons of brown sugar by packing the brown sugar into the measuring spoon and leveling the top of the measuring spoon. Add the packed brown sugar to the stockpot. Stir to combine.

8. Add the apple juice to the stockpot. Stir to combine.

9. Add the puréed frozen squash (substitute puréed canned pumpkin) to the stockpot. Stir to combine. Cover the stockpot with the lid. Increase the heat to medium high until the soup boils then reduce the heat to a gentle simmer. Simmer for 10 minutes to combine flavors.

10. After 10 minutes of simmering add the half-and-half to the stockpot. Stir to combine. Reduce the heat to low and heat the soup to serving temperature. Do not boil or the cream will separate.

11. When the soup is at serving temperature serve immediately with (optional) Gouda or Cheddar cheese on the side.

Italian Vegetable Stew

In summer Italian gardens are abundant with eggplant, tomatoes, bell pepper, and zucchini. This vegetable stew inspired by the bounty of those Italian gardens combines the season's produce with savory herbs and red wine for a hearty, flavorful meal.

Ingredients

1/4 cup olive oil or vegetable oil
1 1/2 cups onion, sliced into crescents
 (about 1/2 of a large onion)
4 cloves garlic, chopped
8 oz mushrooms, washed and sliced
1 red bell pepper, seeded and cut
 into 1/2" strips, strips halved
1 zucchini, ends trimmed,
 halved lengthwise,
 halves sliced into 3/8" thick slices
1 eggplant, peeled and cut into 1" cubes
1 1/2 tsp salt
1/4 tsp black pepper
1/2 tsp thyme, dried
1/2 tsp basil, dried
1/2 tsp marjoram, dried
1/2 tsp rosemary, dried
3/4 tsp oregano, dried
1/4 tsp hot red pepper flakes
1/4 tsp fennel seed, slightly crushed
 (optional)
1 cup red wine
1 bay leaf
1 lb very ripe tomatoes, cut into 1" cubes
 (substitute one 15-oz can tomatoes,
 crushed or diced, do not drain)

Instructions

1. Add the oil to the stockpot. Slice the onion into crescents. Add the onion to the stockpot. Chop the garlic. Add the garlic to the stockpot. Stir to combine. Cook on medium low heat until the onion is soft.

2. While the onion is cooking rinse the mushrooms in the colander and allow them drain thoroughly. Slice the mushrooms. Add the mushrooms to the stockpot. Stir to combine. Increase the heat to medium. Stir occasionally.

3. Wash and seed the bell pepper. Cut the bell pepper into strips 1/2-inch wide. Cut each strip in half. Add the bell pepper to the stockpot. Stir to combine.

4. Wash and trim the ends from the zucchini. Slice the zucchini in half lengthwise. Slice each half into 3/8-inch thick slices. Add the zucchini to the stockpot. Stir to combine.

5. Wash and trim the blossom end from the eggplant. Peel the eggplant. Cut the eggplant into 1-inch cubes. Add the eggplant to the stockpot. Stir to combine.

6. Add the salt, pepper, thyme, basil, marjoram, rosemary, oregano, and red pepper flakes to the small bowl. Stir to combine. Add the mixed seasonings to the stockpot. Stir to combine.

7. If you will be adding the optional fennel seeds then lightly crush them with a mortar and pestle before adding them to the stockpot. If you don't have a mortar and pestle use the back side of a table spoon to crush the fennel seeds against the inside of a small ceramic bowl. You don't need to break apart the seeds, just apply enough pressure to crack the tough seed coating. Lightly crushing the seeds allows their flavor to disperse more quickly.

8. Add the red wine and the bay leaf to the stockpot. Stir to combine.

Continued

Italian Vegetable Stew
- Continued -

Cookware and Utensils

6-quart stockpot with lid
Colander
Vegetable peeler or paring knife
Small bowl
Mortar and pestle or small ceramic bowl
 (if adding the optional fennel seed)

Instructions - continued

9. Wash the tomatoes, cut off the blossom end, and cut them into 1-inch cubes (substitute one 15-oz can crushed or diced tomatoes, undrained). Stir to combine. Cover the stockpot with the lid. Increase the heat to medium high until the stew boils then reduce the heat to a gentle simmer. Simmer covered, stirring occasionally, until the eggplant and zucchini are tender (about 30 minutes).

10. When the eggplant and zucchini are tender remove the bay leaf. Serve the stew hot.

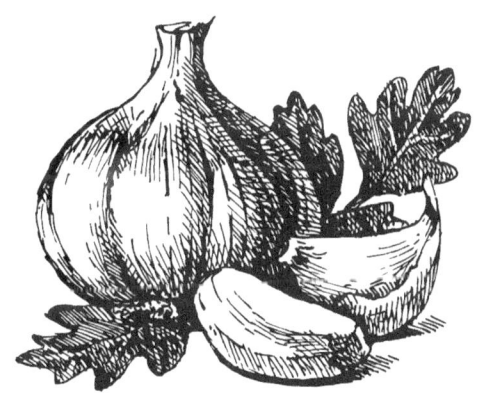

Curry Spiced Lentils

Lentils are a staple in India where meat is expensive and refrigeration is not always available. Dry lentils do not require refrigeration which makes them an ideal substitute for meat in curries. This curried lentil recipe is seasoned with traditional spices to create a vegetarian dish so flavorful and satisfying that non-vegetarians won't miss the meat. These delicious lentils can be served on their own as a stew or add the (optional) shredded Cheddar cheese to serve them as a hot appetizer dip with corn tortilla chips.

Ingredients

1 lb green lentils, dried
6 cups water
1 15-oz can tomato sauce
  (substitute two 8-oz cans tomato sauce)
1 medium onion, finely diced
2 tsp ground coriander
1 tsp ground cumin
1 tsp granulated garlic *
1 TBSP turmeric
1/2 tsp hot red pepper flakes
3/4 tsp cayenne pepper
1/4 tsp ground ginger
1 TBSP mild yellow (sweet)
  curry powder *

For the hot appetizer dip:

2 cups shredded Cheddar cheese *
  (about 8 oz measured by weight)
Corn tortilla chips

* See *Tips* section

Cookware and Utensils

Colander
6-quart stockpot with lid
Small bowl
Shredder/grater (optional)
  (if not using pre-shredded cheese)

Instructions

1. Rinse the lentils in the colander with cold water and allow them to drain thoroughly. Carefully inspect the lentils for rocks or other foreign matter that could chip a tooth and discard if necessary.

2. Add the lentils, 6 cups of water, and the tomato sauce to the stockpot. Stir to combine. Cover the stockpot with the lid. Cook on medium high heat until the lentils begin to boil then reduce the heat to a gentle simmer.

3. While the lentils are cooking finely dice the onion and add it to the stockpot. Stir to combine.

4. Add the coriander, cumin, garlic, turmeric, red pepper flakes, cayenne pepper, ginger, and the curry powder to the small bowl. Stir to combine. Add the seasonings to the stockpot. Stir to combine. Continue simmering the stew, uncovered, until the lentils are soft and mushy (about 20 minutes).

5. When the lentils are cooked you may serve the dish as a stew or continue with the instructions for the hot appetizer dip.

6. To serve as a hot appetizer dip shred the Cheddar cheese and add it to the cooked lentils. Stir to combine. Cover the stockpot with the lid. Adjust the heat to low and heat gently for 5 minutes until the cheese is melted.

7. After the cheese has melted stir the lentils again to evenly disperse the melted cheese. Serve the lentils as a hot appetizer dip with corn tortilla chips.

Vegetables in Season

Spring

Asparagus
Lettuce
Peas
Radishes
Spinach

Summer

Beets
Bell Peppers
Broccoli
Carrots
Celery
Corn
Cucumbers

Eggplant
Garlic
Green Beans
Green Onions
Summer Squash
Tomatoes
Zucchini

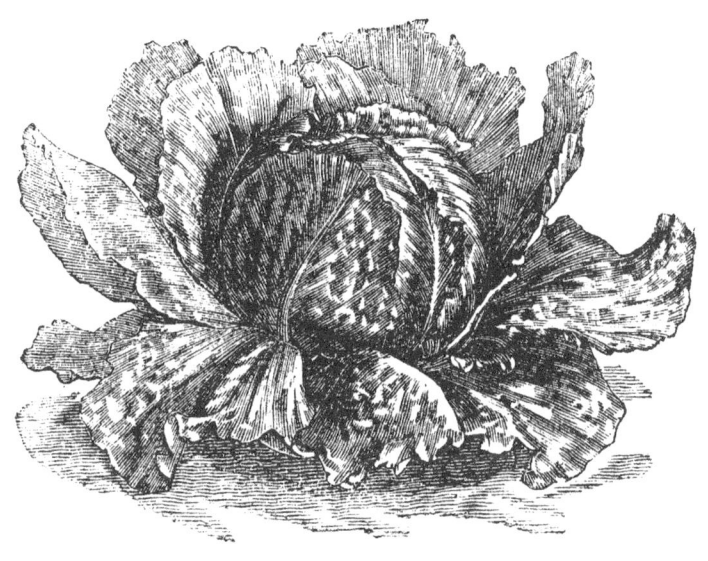

Fall

Broccoli
Cabbage
Carrots
Cauliflower
Garlic
Kale
Onions
Parsnips

Potatoes
Pumpkin
Rutabagas
Sweet Potatoes
Turnips
Winter Squash
Yams

Early Winter

Brussels Sprouts
Cabbage
Kale
Leeks
Onions
Parsnips

Potatoes
Pumpkin
Rutabagas
Sweet Potatoes
Winter Squash
Yams

Photo and Artwork Credits

All graphics and photos courtesy of 123rf.com unless otherwise noted.

Front Cover - Sergii Koval
Back Cover - (courtesy of istockphoto.com) Joem Rynio, knape, PeopleImages
Inside Cover - Daria Ustiugova
Quote - Oleksandr Pakhay, Natalya Levish
Copyright Page - Natalia Hubbert
Dedication - Elena Pimonova
Table of Contents - Natalia Hubbert, Anja Kaiser, Elena Pimonova, Anna Pugach, mykate

Page 1 - Natalya Levish
Page 2 - Johan Larson
Page 3 - Cathy Yeulet / Mark Bowden
Page 4 - choreograph, viewstock
Page 5 - Cathy Yeulet / Mark Bowden
Page 6 - Alisa Katrevich
Page 7 - Nataliia Golovanova
Page 8 - lsantilli
Page 9 - Jochen Schoenfeld
Page 10 - Cathy Yeulet / Mark Bowden
Page 11 - mykate
Page 12 - magone, Heinz Leitner, pretoperola
Page 13 - fedorkondratenko, Roksana Bashyrova
Page 14 - Yuliia Pylypchuk
Page 15 - Evgenii Naumov
Page 16 - Sergiy Kuzmin, Cathy Yeulet / Mark Bowden
Page 17 - belchonock, Valentyn Volkov, Olga Kriger
Page 18 - Marco Mayer, Valentyn Volkov, Sergii Telesh, fpwing
Page 19 - Natallia Khlapushyna, Andrii Gorulko, Vassiliy Prikhodko
Page 20 - oksix
Page 21 - Leigh Anne Meeks, Liv Friis-Larsen
Page 22 - serezniy, magone, Iuliia Burlachenko
Page 23 - homestudio, Georgii Dolgykh, nevodka
Page 24 - Sergejs Rahunoks, givaga
Page 25 - Ingrid Balabanova, Tatjana Baibakova, Milena Lazovic
Page 26 - Amarita Petcharakul, Alexander Raths
Page 27 - Cseh Ioan, Olga Popova
Page 28 - Wavebreak Media Ltd, serezniy,belchonock
Page 29 - Elena Pimonova
Page 30 - kurhan, (graphics by author) Julie Cameron
Page 31 - ifong, Dimitar Sotirov
Page 32 - oksix
Page 33 - ifong, Shvadchak Vasyl
Page 34 - Chris Dorney, squarelogo
Page 35 - serezniy
Page 36 - Sergey Mironov
Page 37 - Yauheniya Litvinovich
Page 38 - (istockphoto.com) DenGuy, BraunS
Page 39 - (istockphoto.com) graletta
Page 40 - Ronnachai Palas
Page 42 - (iStockPhoto.com) Brent Hofacker
Page 43 - Natalia Hubbert
Page 44 - (123rf.com) Dmitrii Kiselev, Oleksandr Chub (istockphoto.com) ra3rn

Page 45 - jirkaejc, Darryl Brooks, Danny Smythe
Page 46 - Aliaksandr Mazurkevich, Jittipong Rakritikul, Dana Bartekoske
Page 47 - Ruslan Kokarev, homestudio, Lasse Kristensen, Sergey Galayko
Page 48 - Igor Terekhov, Ivan Mikhaylov, Andrey Kuzmin
Page 49 - taigi, Konstantin Semenov, Sergey Jarochkin, karandaev
Page 50 - Natalia Hubbert
Page 51 - eshved
Page 52 - myibean, PaylessImages, cloud7days, Penchan Pumila, Alexander Kurlovich
Page 53 - itiir
Page 54 - Anuwat Susomwong, handmadepictures, Roman Tsubin, margouillat
Page 55 - Valter Giumetti, Kitch Bain, Kirill Kirsanov, Ian Allenden
Page 56 - Mona Makela, Marek Uliasz
Page 57 - Natalya Levish
Page 58 - handmadepictures, Brent Hofacker
Page 59 - stocksnapper, Serhiy Hynlosyr
Page 60 - tunedin123
Page 61 - Ivan Dzyuba, Julie Deshaies
Page 62 - Julie Deshaies
Page 63 - Anja Kaiser
Page 77 - alex74
Page 79 - Natalya Levish
Page 83 - Elena Pimonova
Page 91 - Elena Pimonova
Page 94 - mykate
Page 95 to Page 117 - Elena Pimonova
Page 120 - vectorgoods
Page 121 - Anna Pugach
Page 129 - Natalya Levish
Page 135 to Page 149 - Elena Pimonova
Page 151 - alex74
Page 153 to Page 163 - Elena Pimonova
Page 165 - Natalya Levish
Page 167 - Elena Pimonova
Page 168 - qumrran
Page 169 - mykate
Page 173 - Natalya Levish
Page 175 to Page 185 - Elena Pimonova
Page 187 - Patrick Guenette